Pocket Picture Guides

Microbiology of Infectious Diseases

Dilip K. Banerjee
MB BS, MD, PhD, MRC Path
Senior Lecturer in Microbiology
St. George's Hospital Medical School
London, UK.

J.B. Lippincott Company • Philadelphia
Gower Medical Publishing • London • New York

Distributed in USA and Canada by:

J. B. Lippincott Company
East Washington Square
Philadelphia, PA 19105
USA

Distributed in UK and Continental Europe by:

Harper & Row Ltd
Middlesex House
34-42 Cleveland Street
London W1P 5EB
UK

Distributed in Australia and New Zealand by:

Harper & Row (Australasia) Pty Ltd
P.O. Box 226
Artarmon, N.S.W. 2064
Australia

Distributed in Southeast Asia, Hong Kong,
India and Pakistan by:

Harper & Row Publishers (Asia) Pte Ltd
37 Jalan Pemimpin 02-01
Singapore 2057

Distributed in Philippines/Guam, Middle East,
Latin America and Africa by:

Harper & Row International
East Washington Square
Philadelphia, PA 19105
USA

Distribution limited to United Kingdom

ISBN 0-906923-46-8

British Library Cataloguing in Publication Data
Banerjee, Dilip K.
    Microbiology of infectious diseases.–
    (Pocket picture guides to clinical medicine; 6)
    1. Communicable diseases   2. Medical microbiology
    I. Title II. Series
    616.9'041   RC112

Project Editor: Michele Campbell
    Designer: Helen Udesen
    Illustrator: Chris Furey

Reprinted in Hong Kong in 1988

Contents

Acknowledgements
The author would like to thank the following colleagues for providing illustrative material: Dr. J. Almeida, (Fig. 50); Dr. I. Chrystie, St. Thomas' Hospital Medical School, London (Figs. 49, 52, 53, 54, 134); Professor M. A. Epstein/Science Photo Library (Fig. 135); Dr. S. Fisher-Hoch, St. George's Hospital Medical School, London (Fig. 43); Dr. R. Lewis, St. George's Hospital Medical School, London (Figs. 141, 146, 148); Ray Moss, St. George's Hospital Medical School (Figs. 56, 63, 67); Dr. G. Ridgeway, University College Hospital, London (Fig. 121) Professor H. Stern, St. George's Hospital Medical School, London (Figs. 51, 73, 111, 112, 136, 145); Dr. D. C. Warhurst, Hospital for Tropical Diseases, London (Fig. 74).

INTRODUCTION

In this small pocket book an attempt has been made to illustrate pictorially many of the major microbiological causes of infection that we come across in our hospitals and communities. The book does not attempt to provide a comprehensive account of infectious agents and their treatment and should be read in conjunction with a standard text book. However, a ready source of visual information about the common pathogens along with some basic laboratory methods will, I hope, be a valuable guide to clinicians, medical students and laboratory workers. The sections are based on the pattern which is followed in most medical schools for the clinical microbiology course. The reproductions of microscopic illustrations have taken account of the realistic magnification figures, i.e. a bacterial film photographed at a magnification of ×1000 was further enlarged ×2 or ×3 during printing and hence the magnifications in the captions appear larger.

PYOGENIC INFECTIONS

Streptococcal infections *Streptococcus pyogenes*

Description
A Gram-positive spherical organism in short or long chains (Fig. 1), streptococcus causes a variety of pyogenic diseases including follicular tonsillitis, acute sore throat and peritonsillar abscess (quinsy). It also causes pyogenic skin infections like impetigo and cellulitis and generalized septicaemia. Non-pyogenic sequelae viz. rheumatic heart disease and acute glomerulonephritis often follow acute infections of the throat or skin.

Laboratory study
Culture A throat swab taken carefully using a tongue depressor and under well-lit conditions is essential for a positive culture. Culture on blood agar (2% sheep or horse) medium allows rapid isolation and identification. Small transparent colonies with large areas of β-haemolysis grown after overnight incubation are highly characteristic (Fig. 2).

Identification Gram stain of a colony will show typical morphology (Fig. 3). Lancefield's serological method confirms identity and further differentiates streptococci into groups and types. Commercially available modified test reagents are also used for group identification (Fig. 4). Several serological groups have been characterized. Groups A (*Streptococcus pyogenes*), C and G are common causes of throat, respiratory and skin infections. Other groups cause diseases in other parts of the body e.g. group D (enterococci) cause urinary tract infection and group B is commonly associated with neonatal septicaemia and meningitis.

Antibiotic sensitivity
Streptococci are sensitive to a wide variety of antibiotics (Fig. 5) including penicillin (drug of choice), erythromycin, chloramphenicol etc. Group D streptococci are usually resistant to penicillin but sensitive to ampicillin.

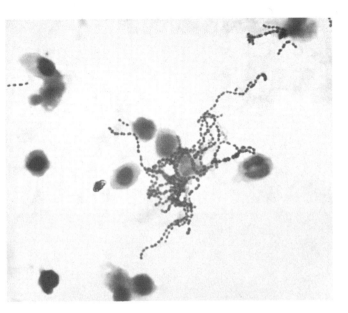

Fig. 1 Gram stain of pus from an empyema cavity showing long and short chains of Gram-positive streptococci and large numbers of pus cells (stained red). *x3,900.*

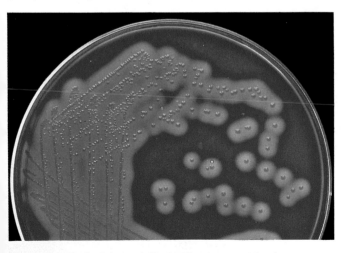

Fig. 2 Growth of a β-haemolytic streptococcus on blood agar medium showing large zones of clear haemolysis around small transparent colonies.

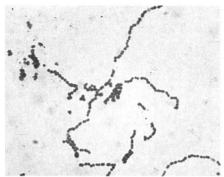

Fig. 3 Smear from a typical β-haemolytic colony. Gram staining shows long and short chains of streptococci. *x2,500*.

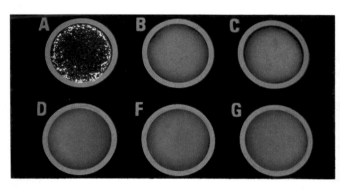

Fig. 4 Modified modern serological grouping method for streptococcus. In this test, latex particles coated with known streptococcal antibodies are mixed with an extract of an unknown streptococcus. Agglutination of the latex particles results if the antigen belongs to the same group as the antibody. This illustration shows a group A positive agglutination test.

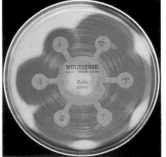

Fig. 5 Antibiotic sensitivity test for streptococcus : *Streptococcus pyogenes* is highly susceptible to a wide variety of common antibiotics including penicillin (P), amoxycillin (AML) and erythromycin (E). The other antibiotics used on this plate are chloramphenicol (C), pipercillin (PRL) and cephradine (CE).

Pyogenic infections of the skin

Common pathogens: *Staphylococcus aureus*
Streptococcus pyogenes

Staphylococcus aureus

Description
Staphylococcus aureus is a Gram-positive coccus,
occurring in clusters (Fig. 6) in pus and it is pathogenic
both at superficial sites as well as in deeper tissues,
including blood. This organism is the commonest cause
of hospital cross-infections. It produces a wide variety of
toxins and enzymes including coagulase. An
enterotoxin-producing staphylococcus causes food
poisoning.

Laboratory study
Culture A swab in transport medium or aspirate (in the
case of abscess) in a sterile bottle is an ideal specimen. A
Gram stain of pus shows clusters of Gram-positive
cocci. Culture on blood agar produces large oil paint-
like pigmented colonies with or without diffuse
haemolysis (Figure 7).
Identification A Gram stained smear shows Gram-
positive cocci (Fig. 8). Confirmation of identity and
pathogenicity is made by a coagulase test. In the slide
coagulase test, human or rabbit plasma is added to a
saline suspension of the organism (Fig. 9 upper). A
positive test produces immediate clumping of the
suspension. The tube coagulase test is performed by
inoculating plasma broth (10% plasma in nutrient
broth) with staphylococci (Fig. 9 left). After 2-4 hours
incubation, a coagulum is formed in a positive test.
(Coagulase negative staphylococci are usually non-
pathogenic except in special situations, e.g. bacterial
endocarditis, urinary tract and hydrocephalus shunt
valves). Bacteriophage typing - see Fig. 10.

Antibiotic sensitivity
Hospital isolates of staphylococci and a large proportion
of community isolates are usually penicillin resistant.
The drug of choice is penicillin in penicillin-sensitive
strains. Cloxacillin (and flucloxacillin), erythromycin,
cephradine, fucidin and lincomycin are some of the
common anti-staphylococcal antibiotics (Fig. 11).

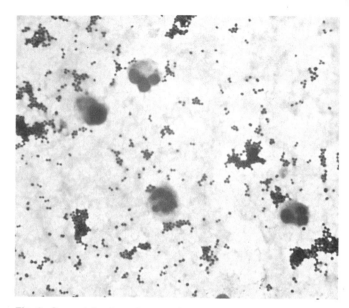

Fig. 6 Gram stain of pus from an abscess, showing clusters of Gram-positive cocci (staphylococci) and Gram-negative pus cells. x3,900.

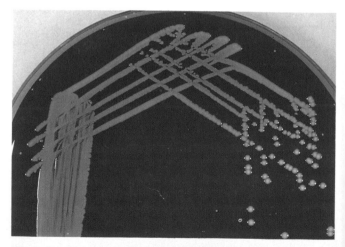

Fig. 7 Growth of staphylococcus on blood agar medium with characteristic pigmentation (golden-yellow) and 'oil paint' appearance.

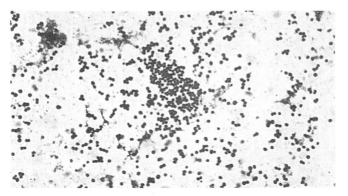

Fig. 8 Gram stained smear of a colony of staphylococcus showing Gram-positive cocci singly and in clusters. *x3,100.*

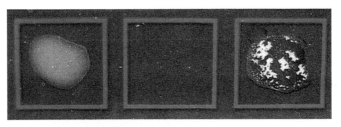

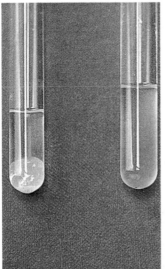

Fig. 9 Coagulase test confirms identity as *Staphylococcus aureus* (coagulase positive) and *Staphylococcus epidermidis* (coagulase negative) :
Slide coagulase test (upper) - when a saline suspension of staphylococci is mixed with human or rabbit plasma on a slide, there is immediate clumping with coagulase positive staphylococci.
Tube coagulase test (left) - when diluted plasma is inoculated with *Staphylococcus aureus*, jellification occurs within 2-4 hrs. This result is due to coagulase converting fibrinogen in the plasma to fibrin and a positive test confirms a positive slide test.

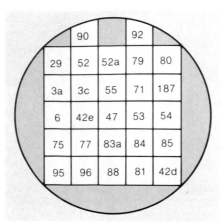

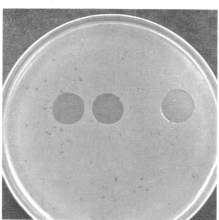

Fig. 10 Bacteriophage typing is used for epidemiological purposes such as locating the source of hospital or community infection. Bacteriophages are bacterial viruses and are used to type bacteria into several phage groups and types. Some phage types are commonly associated with particular types of infection. Typing is done by applying various phage suspensions on a lawn of staphylococcal growth according to the plan shown (upper). After overnight incubation, areas of lysis are produced. The plate shows lysis by phages 52/52A/80 (lower) and this staphylococcus therefore belongs to that phage type - a common hospital epidemic strain.

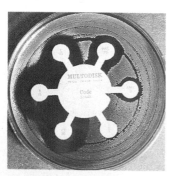

Fig. 11 Antibiotic sensitivity for staphylococcus showing resistance to penicillin - a common finding.

RESPIRATORY INFECTIONS

respiratory infections	
pathogens	**diseases**
Streptococcus pyogenes	acute tonsillitis sore throat
Corynebacterium diphtheriae	diphtheria
Bordetella pertussis	whooping cough
Haemophilus influenzae	acute epiglottitis pneumonia
Streptococcus pneumoniae	pneumonia
Klebsiella pneumoniae *Klebsiella aerogenes* *Pseudomonas aeruginosa* *Staphylococcus aureus*	pneumonia
Legionella pneumophila	pneumonia
Mycobacterium tuberculosis	pulmonary tuberculosis
Mycoplasma pneumoniae	primary atypical pneumonia
Coxiella burnetii	Q fever pneumonia
Chlamydia psittaci	pneumonia
influenza viruses	influenza
respiratory syncytial virus	bronchiolitis
adenovirus coxsackievirus measles virus chickenpox virus	pneumonia
Pneumocystis carinii Aspergillus Candida Cryptococcus Nocardia	opportunistic infection

Diphtheria *Corynebacterium diphtheriae*

Description
A Gram-positive pleomorphic rod sometimes producing the appearance of Chinese letters (Fig. 12). Smears stained by Albert stain (toluidine blue + malachite green) show green rods with dark blue (metachromatic) granules (Fig. 13). Infection by this organism results in pseudomembrane formation in the throat, pharynx, larynx, nose, conjunctiva and sometimes in the vagina in young children. A powerful exotoxin is produced locally which, when absorbed, causes myocardial damage and also affects nerves, kidneys and adrenals.

Laboratory study
Culture A throat swab or preferably a small piece of pseudomembrane will show characteristic organisms on staining. Culture on tellurite-containing medium produces characteristic growth (Fig. 14). Three morphological varieties are identifiable - *gravis*, *intermedius* and *mitis*.

Identification Gram or Albert stains show the typical morphology. A serum-sugar fermentation test identifies the pathogenic forms. A toxigenicity test confirms the virulence property. This is done by the Elek plate virulence test (Fig. 15). A diphtheria antitoxin-soaked blotting paper strip is sunk in melted agar. After the agar is set, bacterial inoculum is streaked at right angles to the paper strip. After 24-48 hrs incubation, the plates are examined for precipitation lines. Known toxin-producing and toxin-negative strains are included as controls. The precipitation lines of the test strain join up with the lines produced by the toxin-positive strain (reaction of identity) if the toxins are identical, thereby confirming the identity of the test strain as a toxigenic strain. All three varieties can be toxigenic although *gravis* is generally considered to be the most virulent.

Antibiotic sensitivity
Generally *Corynebacterium diphtheriae* is very sensitive to most antibiotics (Fig. 16). Penicillin and erythromycin are most effective in the treatment of diphtheria along with diphtheria antitoxin.

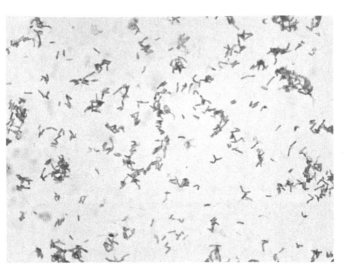

Fig. 12 Gram stained smear of *Corynebacterium diphtheriae* showing Gram-positive pleomorphic rods and Chinese letter arrangements. *x3,000.*

Fig. 13 Albert stain of *C. diphtheriae* showing green rods and typical dark blue metachromatic granules. *x3,100.*

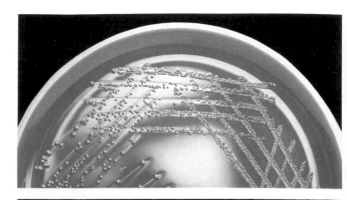

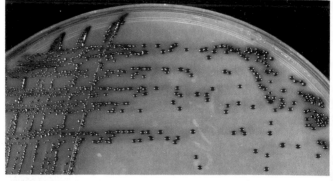

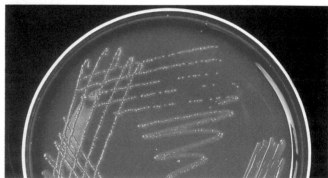

Fig. 14 Growth of *C. diphtheriae* colonies on:
a tellurite-containing medium, producing black colonies.
b Tinsdale medium, producing characteristic haloes around the colonies.
c blood agar plate, producing uncharacteristic colonies.

11

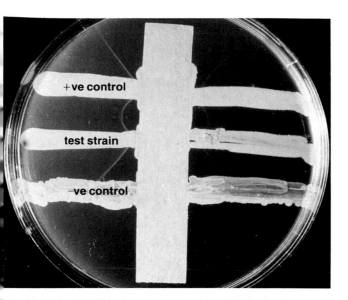

Fig. 15 Elek plate. This demonstrates toxin production by *C. diphtheriae*.

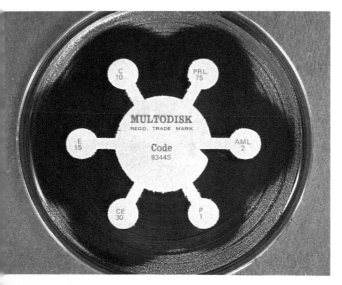

Fig. 16 Antibiotic sensitivity test for *C. diphtheriae*, which is susceptible to a variety of antibiotics.

Whooping cough

Common pathogens: *Bordetella pertussis*
Bordetella parapertussis (only 2% cases)

Description
A short Gram-negative (parvobacterium) rod (Fig. 17),
found in the secretions of the upper respiratory tract in
the catarrhal and early 'whoop' stage of the disease,
which almost exclusively occurs in infants and small
children.

Laboratory study
Culture A pernasal swab taken with meticulous care is
absolutely essential (Fig. 18). Cough plates (culture
plates exposed near the patient's mouth during a cough-
ing bout) are not always rewarding. The swab is transported, preferably in a special transport medium containing charcoal, and is cultured onto a Bordet-Gengou
medium (or a modification of it) which contains 20-
30% blood and penicillin. Growth of mercury-drop or
half pearl-like colonies after 24-48 hrs incubation is
characteristic (Fig. 19).
Identification This is done by a slide agglutination test
with specific antisera. Type 1:3 is currently the common
pathogenic variety in Britain, but is changeable.

Antibiotic sensitivity
Bordetella is generally very sensitive, but antibiotic
treatment is of limited value. Infectivity is highest during the early catarrhal stage of the disease and gradually
declines as the patient shows symptoms of 'whoop'.
Antibiotic treatment is of some value in the reduction of
spread to immediate contacts.

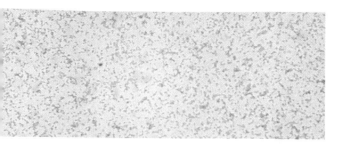

Fig. 17 Gram stained smear of *Bordetella pertussis* showing short Gram-negative rods. *x3,200.*

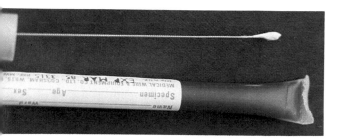

Fig. 18 A pernasal swab - a thin malleable wire with a small cottonwool wisp. The swab is gently passed through the anterior nares, quickly twisted and withdrawn and transported immediately to the laboratory in transport medium containing charcoal.

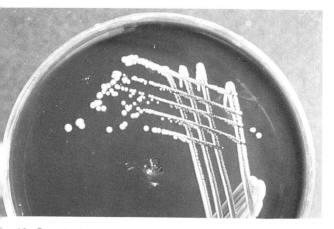

Fig. 19 Growth of *Bordetella pertussis* on charcoal- containing medium showing 'mercury drop' colonies.

Description
A short Gram-negative bacillus with very
fastidious growth requirements (Fig. 20), this organism
causes a variety of clinical diseases including acute
epiglottitis, pneumonia, otitis media, conjunctivitis,
acute pyogenic meningitis and arthritis.

Laboratory study
Culture Freshly coughed-up sputum collected in a
wide-mouthed bottle and free from saliva (as far as is
practicable), or bronchial aspirate are suitable specimens. In acute epiglottitis, utmost care should be taken
to collect a swab. The specimen should be cultured on
blood-containing media. Whole blood agar is inade-
quate but lysed blood or chocolate agar allows luxuriant
growth (Fig. 21). Whole blood provides factor X
(haematin) whereas factor V (NADPH - a nucleic acid
product) is released from inside the blood cells when
blood is laked. Both these factors are essential for
growth of *Haemophilus*.
Identification This can be confirmed by the demonstration of requirement for the above factors. A nutrient
agar plate is inoculated with the organism and filter
paper discs containing X, V and XV factors are
implanted on the inoculated plates. After overnight
incubation, growth is seen around the disc containing
both factors but not around X or V factors alone (Fig.
22). *Haemophilus parainfluenzae*, a less virulent organism, requires only V factor and will therefore grow
around both V and XV discs. The identity of *Haemophilus influenzae* can be further confirmed by the 'satellitism' test (Fig. 23) and by a slide agglutination test
with specific antisera. Several types of the organism are
described, type B being the most virulent.

Antibiotic sensitivity
H. influenzae is generally sensitive to many antibiotics
(Fig. 24). The drug of choice for treatment is ampicillin,
although resistance to this drug has increased in recent
years. Erythromycin and chloramphenicol are also very
effective. Chloramphenicol is favoured by some for
treatment of meningitis due to *H. influenzae*, especially
because it diffuses better.

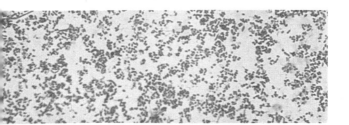

Fig. 20 Gram stained smear of *Haemophilus influenzae* showing small Gram-negative rods. *x3,700.*

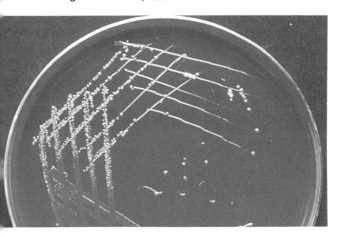

Fig. 21 Growth of *Haemophilus influenzae* on chocolate agar medium.

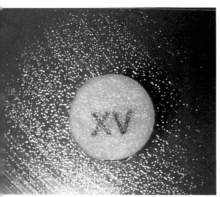

Fig. 22 Test to show special growth requirement of *H. influenzae*. It requires X(haematin) and V(NADPH) factors for its growth. A nutrient agar plate inoculated with this organism will fail to support growth except in the immediate vicinity of a disc containing both the factors.

16

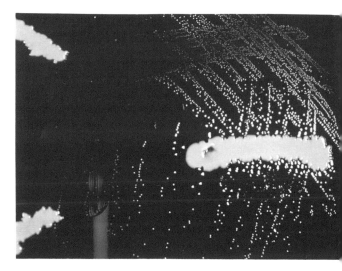

Fig. 23 'Satellitism' test : in this test, growth of *H. influenzae* occurs around a staphylococcus colony (providing V factor) on a blood agar plate (blood provides H factor but not V unless laked. Blood agar plates contain whole blood).

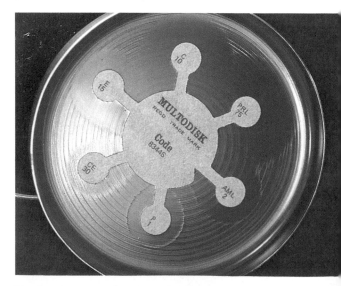

Fig. 24 Antibiotic sensitivity of *H. influenzae* on chocolate agar medium. There is general sensitivity to a wide variety of antibiotics.

Streptococcus pneumoniae
(Pneumococcus or *Diplococcus pneumoniae*)

Description
A Gram-positive, lanceolate-shaped diplococcus
usually with a large capsule in virulent types, it
is a common cause of acute lobar pneumonia (Fig. 25).
Streptococcus pneumoniae also causes broncho-
pneumonia, lung abscess, empyema, meningitis, septicaemia and infection of the middle ear and eyes.

Laboratory study
Culture Freshly coughed-up sputum of characteristic
'rusty' appearance shows masses of typical cocci on
Gram staining (Fig. 26). Culture on blood or chocolate
agar (preferably in 5% CO_2) shows small α-haemolytic
'draughtsman' type colonies with concentric rings (Fig.
27). Virulent forms often produce mucoid colonies.
Identification These are identified by colony appearance and microscopic morphology and by the optochin
sensitivity test. Optochin (ethyl hydrocuprein) is inhibitory to pneumococcus but not to normal, non-
pathogenic, mouth flora, *Streptococcus viridans*, which
also grows abundantly from sputum as α-haemolytic
colonies (Fig. 28). Other methods of confirmation are
also available but are not very commonly used. Several
serological types of pneumococci are identifiable, some
more often from human infections e.g. type 3 in acute
lobar pneumonia and meningitis.
  Demonstration of pneumococcal antigen in the
sputum (or in CSF in pneumococcal meningitis) by the
counterimmunoelectrophoresis technique using polyvalent anti-pneumococcal serum may give a quick
diagnosis (see Fig. 110).

Antibiotic sensitivity
Pneumococci are generally very sensitive to common
antibiotics (Fig. 29). Penicillin is the drug of choice,
alternatively erythromycin, co-trimoxazole or a cephalosporin may be used.

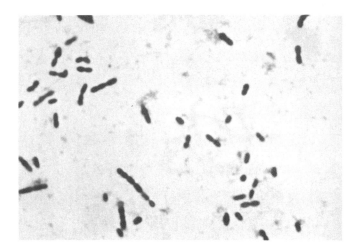

Fig. 25 Gram stained film of pneumococci, showing Gram-positive lanceolate diplococci. *x3,100*.

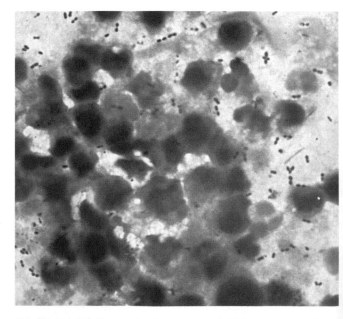

Fig. 26 Gram stain of sputum from a patient with lobar pneumonia, showing large numbers of Gram-positive lanceolate diplococci and pus cells. *x3,500*.

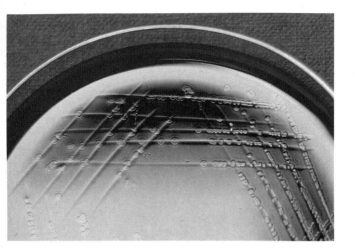

Fig. 27 Growth of pneumococci on blood agar showing characteristic 'draughtsman' colonies with concentric surface rings.

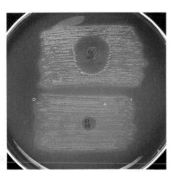

Fig. 28 Optochin sensitivity of pneumococci in contrast with *Streptococcus viridans* which also produces α-haemolytic colonies on blood agar.

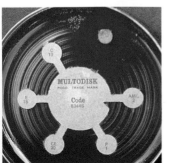

Fig. 29 Antibiotic sensitivity of pneumococci. These are generally very sensitive to common antibiotics.

20

Klebsiella spp.

Description
These are thick Gram-negative rods of low pathogenicity, but can cause severe infection in old age, postoperatively and as opportunist infections (Fig. 30).

Laboratory study
Culture *Klebsiella* grows well on common media (Fig. 31); large, weakly lactose-fermenting mucoid colonies are produced on MacConkey's medium (Fig. 32).
Identification is confirmed by morphology (Fig. 33) and biochemical tests.

Antibiotic sensitivity
Klebsiella species are resistant to common antibiotics (Fig. 34). If treatment is indicated, a new cephalosporin with or without gentamicin is an effective regimen.

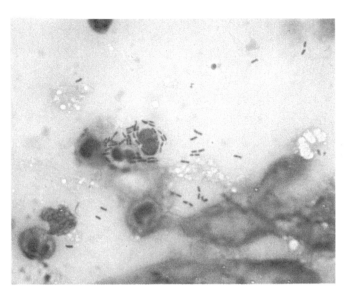

Fig. 30 Gram stained smear of sputum from a chronic bronchitic, showing thick, stout Gram-negative rods of the predominant organism - *Klebsiella*. x3,000.

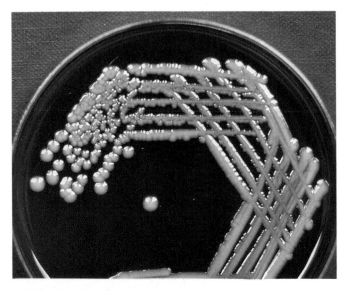

Fig. 31 Growth of very mucoid *Klebsiella* colonies on blood agar.

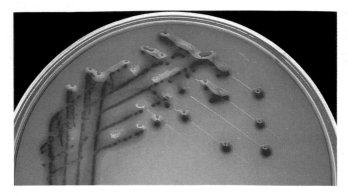

Fig. 32 Growth of *Klebsiella* on MacConkey's medium showing lactose-fermenting, very mucoid colonies.

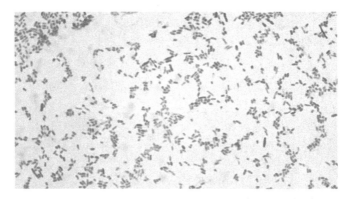

Fig. 33 Gram stained smear from a *Klebsiella* culture showing large, thick Gram-negative rods. *x2,400.*

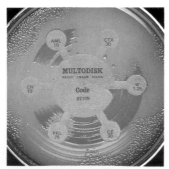

Fig. 34 Antibiotic sensitivity of *Klebsiella* showing unusual resistance to a number of antibiotics.

Pseudomonas spp.

Description
These are long slender Gram-negative rods of
doubtful pathogenicity, but may be associated
with fulminating infection, particularly septicaemia, as
an opportunist infection.

Laboratory study
Culture Purulent sputum on culture yields greenish
pigment-producing colonies on most common media
(Figs. 35 and 36). Non-lactose fermenting colonies with
a metallic sheen and dark green pigmentation are
usually produced on MacConkey's medium (Fig. 37).
Identification is confirmed by morphology (Fig. 38),
the oxidase test [tetramethyl-paraphenylene diamine
dihydrochloride (Fig. 39) - positive only with
Pseudomonas and *Neisseria*] and biochemical tests (not
always required).

Antibiotic sensitivity
Pseudomonas species are resistant to common antibiotics. Anti-pseudomonal antibiotics (gentamicin,
amikacin, carbenicillin, pipercillin and colistin) are
usually required singly or in combination (Fig. 40).

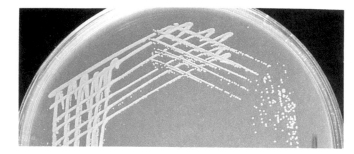

Fig. 35 Growth of *Pseudomonas* on nutrient agar medium.

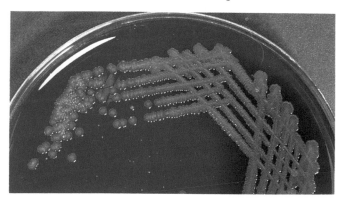

Fig. 36 *Pseudomonas* culture on blood agar medium.

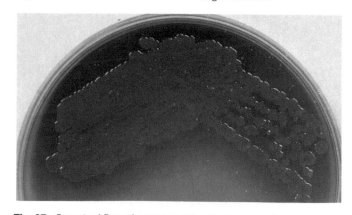

Fig. 37 Growth of *Pseudomonas* on MacConkey's medium showing dark green pigment.

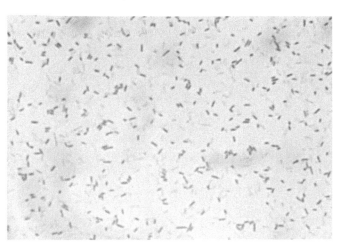

Fig. 38 Gram stained film of *Pseudomonas* showing long, slender Gram-negative rods. *x3,900.*

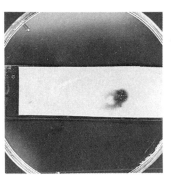

Fig. 39 Oxidase test - positive reaction with formation of purple colour.

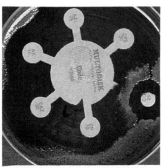

Fig. 40 Sensitivity of *Pseudomonas* to anti-pseudomonal antibiotics.

Description
This is a small Gram-negative rod of unusual pathogen-icity (Fig. 41). It is an environmental organism of ubiquitous distribution - found in water, both domestic supply and natural, and has been thought to withstand temperatures of up to about 55°C. *L. pneumophila* has been incriminated as the cause of a number of outbreaks of acute severe to mild respiratory illnesses resembling atypical pneumonia.

Laboratory study
Culture Material from the patient (usually sputum, bronchial aspirate or pieces of post-mortem lung tissue) or water from suspected sites are cultured on a special selective medium (charcoal yeast extract) containing various antibiotics (Fig. 42). Isolation is not always easy. The immunofluorescence technique may be help-ful for indicating the presence of the organism in clinical material as well as being used for the detection of antibody in the patient's blood (Fig. 43).
Identification is usually by serological methods.

Antibiotic sensitivity
This is not usually necessary. These organisms are usually sensitive to erythromycin and rifampicin.

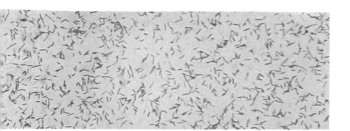

Fig. 41 Gram stained smear of *Legionella pneumophila*, counter-stained with carbol fuchsin, showing slender Gram-negative rods. *x3,900.*

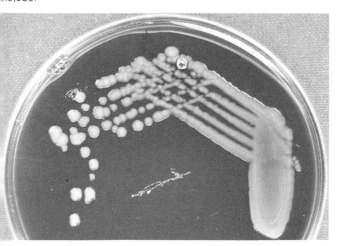

Fig. 42 Growth of *L. pneumophila* on selective charcoal-containing medium.

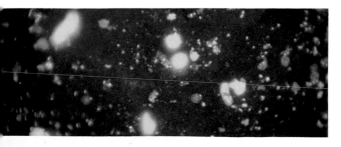

Fig. 43 Immunofluorescent staining of *L. pneumophila* in the bronchial aspirate. *x2,700.*

Description

Beaded acid-fast bacilli (Fig. 44) of high virulence causing tuberculous disease of the lung commonly and also of the lymph nodes, meninges, kidneys, bone and joints and occasionally at other sites.

Laboratory study

Culture Since about 95% of infections are pulmonary, sputum is the main clinical specimen. Other specimens include CSF, lymph node and tissue biopsies, aspirates from the pleural cavity and other cavities including joints, urine etc. The specimen is cultured on Löwenstein-Jensen medium after appropriate decontamination (the medium contains egg, mineral salts and malachite green) and is incubated for 4-8 weeks. Growth appears after about 4 weeks incubation as granular buff-coloured colonies (Fig. 45). Some atypical mycobacteria (usually opportunists) produce colonies of different morphology and colour (Fig. 46). **Identification** This is made by acid-fast stained morphology (Fig. 47), fluorochrome staining (Fig. 48) and special tests e.g. the niacin test (positive for *M. tuberculosis* and negative for *M. bovis*) which is usually done in a reference laboratory.

Antibiotic sensitivity

Löwenstein-Jensen medium containing various concentrations of antibiotics is used to test the sensitivity of the isolates. Common antibiotics used are isoniazid, rifampicin, ethambutol, streptomycin and pyrazinamide.

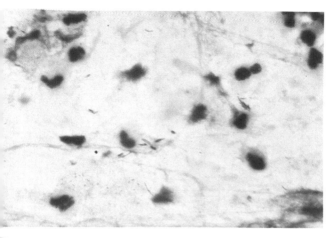

Fig. 44 Smear of sputum with Ziehl-Neelsen stain, showing acid-fast beaded bacilli in a background of tissue debris and non acid-fast bacteria (stained blue with methylene blue counterstain). *x2,800.*

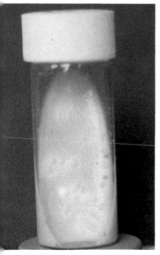

Fig. 45 Growth of mycobacteria on Löwenstein-Jensen medium after four weeks incubation. Rough, buff-coloured colonies are characteristic of *M. tuberculosis*.

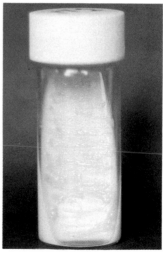

Fig. 46 Growth of atypical mycobacteria - *M. kansasii* with distinct yellow pigment.

30

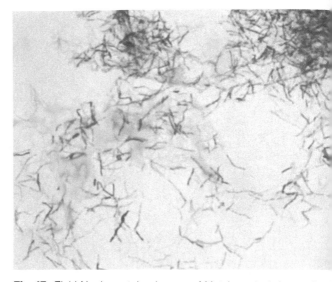

Fig. 47 Ziehl-Neelsen stained smear of *M. tuberculosis* from culture showing beaded acid-fast bacilli. x3,000.

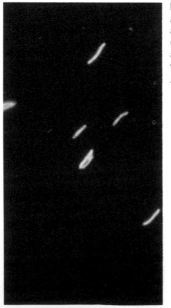

Fig. 48 Fluorochrome stain of *M. tuberculosis* with a mixture of auramine O and rhodamine B (Truant stain). Mycobacteria appeàr fluorescent when viewed under ultraviolet light. x3,500.

31

Clinical features

Viruses are responsible for the majority of infections of the respiratory tract. Such infections are generally mild and are usually caused by rhino- (Fig. 49) and corona- (Fig. 50) viruses and occasionally by adenoviruses (Fig. 51), parainfluenza (Fig. 52) and enteroviruses. Viral pneumonia is caused predominantly by influenza viruses (Fig. 53) although parainfluenza, adenoviruses, measles and chickenpox viruses have sometimes been responsible. Infantile bronchiolitis is caused almost exclusively by respiratory syncytial virus (Fig. 54).

Laboratory diagnosis

The practical value of the diagnosis of viral respiratory diseases is doubtful, because of the short and mild nature of the clinical disease and the time-consuming and expensive diagnostic techniques. Viruses can be isolated from secretions from the respiratory tract e.g. nasal and throat washings and swabs (transported to the laboratory without delay). Paired sera for viral antibodies provide valuable retrospective information and may be of great value in epidemiological investigations.

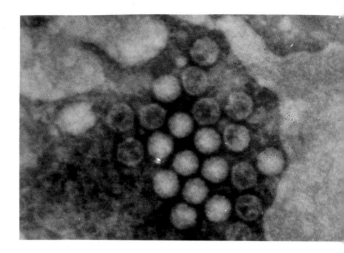

Fig.49 Rhinovirus. A small RNA virus, having a similar electron-micrographic structure and size (20 - 30 nm) to an enterovirus, this is a major cause of the common cold in all age groups. Over 100 serotypes have now been distinguished. These are cultured in human and monkey cell cultures at 33°C (approximately the temperature of the nose). *x273,600*.

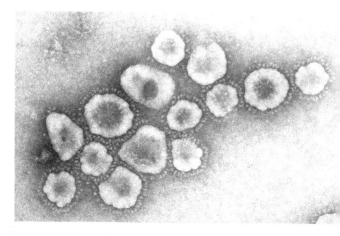

Fig. 50 Electronmicrograph of coronaviruses. These are small RNA viruses (80 - 160 nm in diameter) with an ill-defined nucleocapsid core, around which petal-shaped peplomeres are arranged. This virus is a frequent cause of the common cold in man. *x78,800*

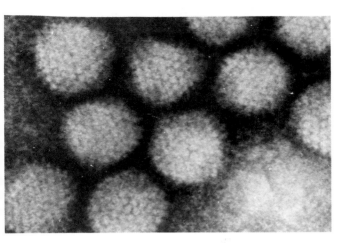

Fig. 51 Electronmicrograph of an adenovirus; an important cause of acute viral respiratory disease. The virus particles are about 60-90 nm in diameter and have a dense, central DNA core and an ornate icosahedral outer capsid composed of particles (capsomeres). x293,100.

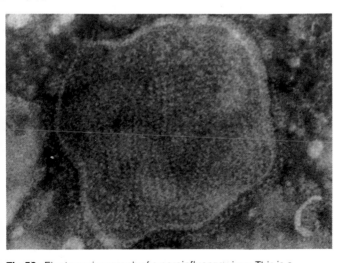

Fig.52 Electronmicrograph of a parainfluenza virus. This is a member of the paramyxovirus family, which also includes mumps, measles and respiratory syncytial virus. The virions are 125 - 250 nm in diameter and are surrounded by an envelope which is covered with spikes and rods (haemagglutinin and neuraminidase). The core contains filamentous nucleocapsids. x258,000.

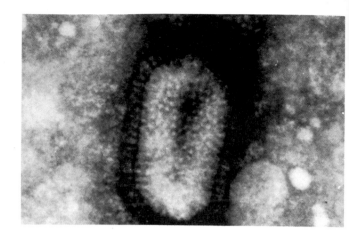

Fig.53 Electronmicrograph of influenza virus. This is a member of the orthomyxovirus family. It is similar in structure to, but smaller than, the paramyxoviruses, being 80 - 120 nm in diameter. The virions are roughly spherical, and surrounded by an envelope which contains radially-projecting spikes of virus haemagglutinin and neuraminidase. *x273,000.*

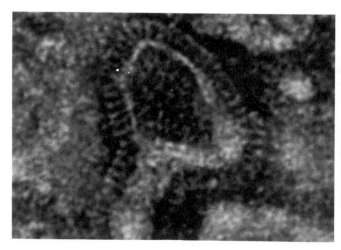

Fig. 54 Respiratory syncytial virus (RSV) is an enveloped RNA virus belonging to the paramyxovirus group and is the commonest cause of infantile respiratory disease, especially bronchiolitis. In cell cultures the RSV causes cell fusion and syncytium formation, and hence is so called. Immunofluorescence tests for viral antigen in the nasopharyngeal cells can be used for rapid diagnosis. *x273,000.*

GASTRO-INTESTINAL INFECTIONS

gastro-intestinal infections	
common pathogens	**diseases**
bacterial	
Salmonella (human)	typhoid and other enteric fevers
Salmonella (animal)	food poisoning
Shigella	dysentery
Vibrio	cholera
Campylobacter	enterocolitis
E. coli	infantile gastro-enteritis travellers' diarrhoea
Yersinia	enterocolitis
parasitic	
Giardia	diarrhoea tropical sprue
Entamoeba	amoebic dysentery
helminths	diarrhoea and other manifestations
viral	
rotavirus	viral diarrhoea
enteroviruses	winter vomiting disease viral diarrhoea

Typhoid and other enteric infections

Common pathogens: *Salmonella typhi*
Salmonella paratyphi A, B and C

Description
Salmonella organisms are Gram-negative bacilli of high virulence and pathogenicity (Fig. 55). They are highly motile with flagella all round them - peritrichous flagella (Fig. 56). All the above varieties cause enteric fevers but *S. typhi* causes more severe infection with prominent systemic manifestations and moderate to severe intestinal effects.

Laboratory study
Culture Isolation of the organisms can be made from blood, faeces and urine samples during various stages of the disease. They grow readily on ordinary media but a selective medium like DCA or SS allows quicker and easier isolation (Figs. 57 and 58). The isolates from clinical specimens are identified by slide agglutination with specific antisera (commercially available) and by a battery of biochemical tests. API is a modern and simple biochemical test system (Fig. 59). Identification is further confirmed by detecting antibody (Widal test) in the patient's blood against somatic O, flagellar H and capsular Vi antigens of the organisms (Figure 60). A progressive increase in the titre of antibody at various stages of the disease strongly suggests current infection.

Antibiotic sensitivity
These organisms are generally sensitive to a wide variety of antibiotics including chloramphenicol, ampicillin and septrin - the three antibiotics most commonly used against this infection (Fig. 61).

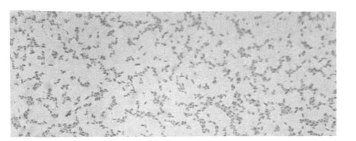

Fig. 55 Gram stained smear of *Salmonella typhi* showing Gram-negative, rod-shaped organisms. *x2,600.*

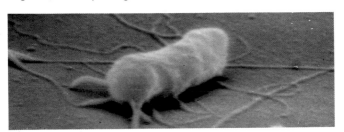

Fig. 56 Scanning electronmicrograph of *Salmonella* showing peritrichous flagella. *x18,000.*

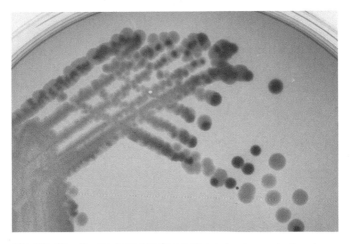

Fig. 57 Growth of lactose non-fermenting colourless colonies of *Salmonella* on MacConkey's medium. Lactose fermenting *E. coli* and *Streptococcus faecalis* also grew from this faecal specimen as commensal gut organisms.

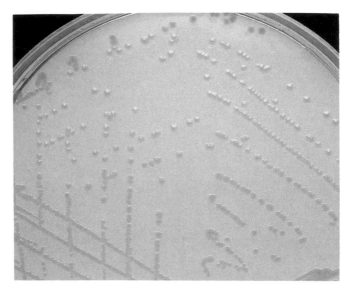

Fig. 58 Growth of *Salmonella* on selective DCA (deoxycholate citrate agar) medium, on which some non-pathogenic gut commensals are inhibited from growing.

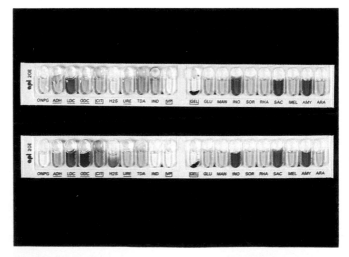

Fig. 59 Biochemical identification of *Salmonella* by the API test (bottom). A parallel test with *E. coli* is also shown for comparison (top).

widal test	serum dilutions								
antigens	$\frac{1}{20}$	$\frac{1}{40}$	$\frac{1}{80}$	$\frac{1}{160}$	$\frac{1}{320}$	$\frac{1}{640}$	$\frac{1}{1280}$	$\frac{1}{2560}$	control
S. typhi O	+	+	+	+	−	−	−	−	−
S. typhi H	+	+	+	+	+	+	+	−	−
S. paratyphi B H	−	−	−	−	−	−	−	−	−
S. paratyphi B O	+a	+a	−	−	−	−	−	−	−

+ = indicates agglutination
a = weak response probably due to antigenic cross-reactivity

Fig. 60 Widal test to detect typhoid antibody in patient's blood. A representative result, twelve days after the onset of the illness, shows high levels of antibody to both somatic O and flagellar H antigens of *S. typhi*. Seven days after the onset there was a weak positive response to *S. typhi* H antigen up to 1/80 dilution. A strong positive response to O antigen has more diagnostic significance. Other antigens, viz *S. paratyphi* A may be included in the test if there is a suggestive history (e.g. travel in endemic areas).

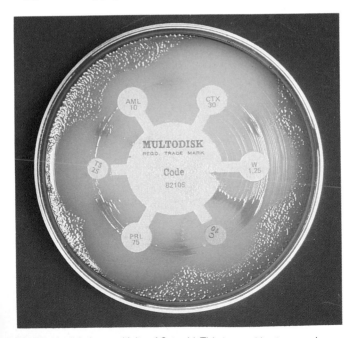

Fig.61 Antibiotic sensitivity of *S. typhi*. This is sensitive to a number of antibiotics including chloramphenicol, ampicillin and co-trimoxazole - the drugs of choice for the treatment of this infection.

Dysentery

Common pathogens: *Shigella dysenteriae*
Shigella flexneri   *Shigella boydii*   *Shigella sonnei*

Description
These are Gram-negative organisms of
moderate to severe virulence (Figs. 62 and 63). *Shigella sonnei* is the commonest species found in the developed world and causes mild diarrhoea, usually amongst institutionalized patients, and particularly in homes for the mentally retarded and geriatric hospitals. Other *Shigella* organisms are found more commonly in less developed parts of the world and cause more acute manifestations including severe dehydration.

Laboratory study
Culture Isolation of these organisms from faecal samples is reasonably easy, especially when a selective medium like DCA or an enrichment medium like selinite F is employed for primary culture.
Identification The non lactose-fermenting (colourless) colonies on MacConkey's medium (Fig. 64) and DCA (Fig. 65) are identified by slide agglutination with specific antisera and by biochemical tests (using an API or an alternative system).

Antibiotic sensitivity
Shigella organisms are very sensitive to the antibiotics used for gut infections (Fig. 66). In the majority of infections no antibiotic treatment is required, and fluid replacement alone may be sufficient. In some acute infections, however, particularly those caused by *Shigella dysenteriae*, antibiotic treatment in addition to fluid replacement may be necessary. In these situations an appropriate antibiotic like ampicillin, septrin or a non-absorbable sulpha may be used.

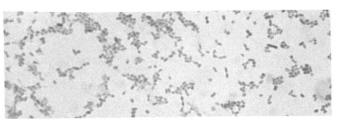

Fig. 62 Gram stained film of *Shigella* showing Gram-negative rods. *x3,300.*

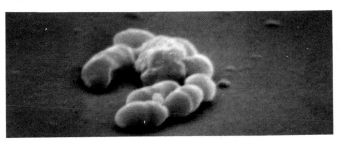

Fig. 63 Scanning electronmicrograph of *Shigella* showing aflagellar morphology. These are non-motile organisms. *x12,300.*

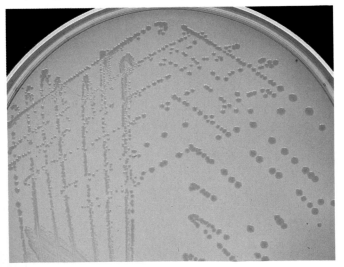

Fig. 64 Growth of *Shigella* on MacConkey's medium, showing colourless lactose non-fermenting colonies.

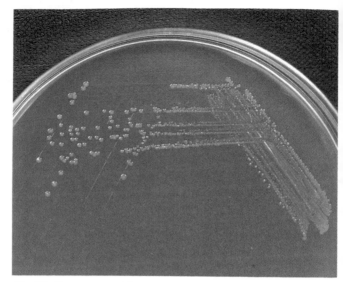

Fig. 65 Pure growth of *Shigella* on DCA medium.

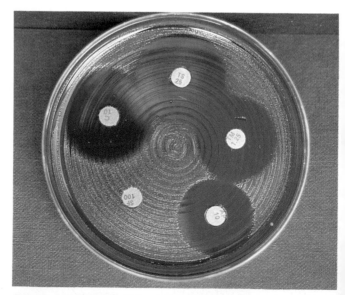

Fig. 66 Antibiotic sensitivity of *Shigella* showing sulphonamide resistance.

Food poisoning

Clinical varieties	Pathogens involved
Toxic - due to absorption from the gut of a ready-made toxin in the food. (enterotoxin)	
Some usually present as vomiting, abdominal pain and diarrhoea a few hours (2-6) after the intake of food.	*Staphylococcus aureus* *Bacillus cereus*
Others present predominantly with symptoms of neurological involvement with motor paralysis.	*Clostridium botulinum*
Toxic and invasive	*Clostridium perfringens*
Invasive - due to multiplication of the organisms in the gut in large numbers.	
The usual manifestations are diarrhoea, abdominal pain and sometimes vomiting starting much later (8-24 hrs) after ingestion of infected food.	*Clostridium perfringens* *Salmonella typhimurium*

Laboratory study
Culture Isolation of the responsible agents from food, faeces and vomitus can be made by employing appropriate techniques. In the toxic type, toxin can be detected in the patient's blood and in food by immuno-diffusion and other techniques.

Epidemiological investigation in collaboration with public health personnel is important in order to locate the source and prevent further outbreaks.

Antibiotic sensitivity
This is not required. Antibiotic treatment is not necessary but in acute cases replenishment of fluid is essential.

Cholera

Common pathogens: *Vibrio cholerae* biotype El Tor
Vibrio cholerae biotype classical

Description
A highly motile (Fig. 67), weakly Gram-negative,
curved (comma-shaped) organism (Fig. 68), this has
previously been the cause of high mortality and enor-
mous disability worldwide and is still a major public
health problem in the developing world. The infection is
clinically manifested by profuse 'rice-water' diarrhoea,
dehydration and the consequences of the latter. A
potent exotoxin is responsible for the pathophysiological
changes in the intestinal mucus membrane leading to
massive fluid and electrolyte loss.

Laboratory study
Culture Faecal specimens cultured on ordinary media
would allow growth of the vibrios but special media like
TCBS (thiosulphate, citrate, bile salt and sucrose) agar
allows selective isolation of the organisms in pure culture (Fig. 69). Preliminary enrichment in alkaline pep-
tone water sometimes enhances the isolation rate.
Identification Biochemical and serological tests with
specific antisera (slide agglutination) allow identification of the isolates. There are special biochemical
tests to differentiate between classical and El Tor bio-
types. The El Tor biotype is now the predominant
organism in endemic areas.

Antibiotic sensitivity
Vibrio cholerae is sensitive to a number of common
antibiotics (Fig. 70). Antibiotics are not commonly
required for treatment of cholera. Rehydration with
fluid and replenishment of electrolytes is the mainstay
of treatment.

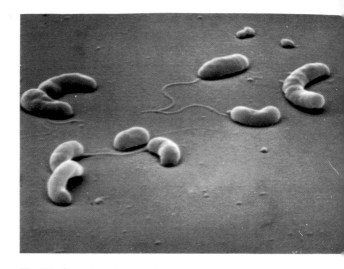

Fig. 67 Scanning electronmicrograph of *Vibrio cholerae* showing single polar flagellum. *x13,000*.

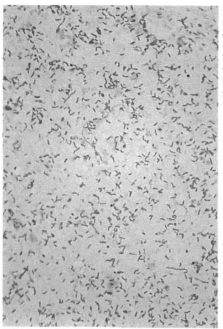

Fig. 68 Gram stained morphology of *Vibrio* with many comma-shaped bacilli. The smear was counterstained by dilute carbol fuchsin. *x3,900*.

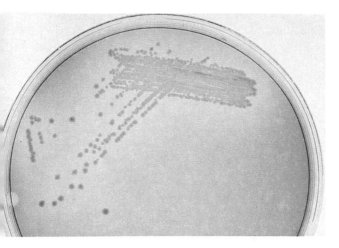

Fig. 69 Growth of *Vibrio* on TCBS medium. *Vibrio cholerae* produces yellow colonies on this selective medium.

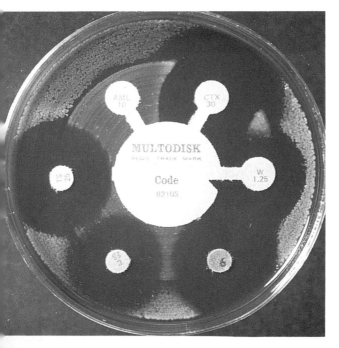

Fig. 70 Antibiotic sensitivity of *Vibrio cholerae*

48

Campylobacter diarrhoea

Common pathogens: *Campylobacter jejuni*
Campylobacter coli

Description
An actively motile, curved, Gram-negative organism, this is probably the most important cause of diarrhoea in Britain (Fig 71). It is a water- and milk-borne infection and is transmitted from infected animals (cattle, dogs, poultry) which probably act as a reservoir of infection. Characteristic clinical features include abdominal pain, diarrhoea with blood and mucus, fever and body ache.

Laboratory study
Culture *Campylobacter* species are fastidious in their growth requirements and prefer a microaerophilic environment. Ten percent CO_2, reduced oxygen and a higher temperature (41°C) in addition to added antibiotics (vancomycin, trimethoprim and polymixin - to inhibit commensals) allow selective growth of these organisms from diarrhoeal faeces (Fig. 72).
Identification Characteristic growth in the above environment confirms the identity of these organisms. Further confirmation is made by motility and a Gram stain.

Antibiotic sensitivity
Erythromycin is the drug of choice and nearly all strains are sensitive to this.

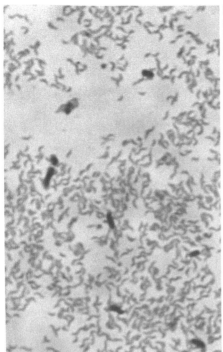

Fig. 71 Gram stained film of *Campylobacter* with dilute carbol fuchsin counterstain. Various characteristic arrangements can be seen including 'gull-wing', 'S' and spiral forms. *x3,700*.

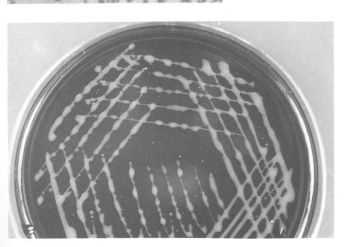

Fig. 72 Growth of *Campylobacter* on special medium, incubated in a special environment.

50

Viral diarrhoea

Description
Viruses are often responsible for diarrhoea both in children and in adults. Vomiting is usually a common feature and in severe cases, dehydration may result. The infection spreads rapidly within families and institutions and is usually self-resolving. Rehydration may be necessary in severe cases. Rotavirus (Fig. 73), belonging to the reovirus group, is the commonest cause of viral diarrhoea but viruses like winter vomiting disease virus and Norwalk agents have also been known to cause diarrhoea both in children and in adults.

Laboratory study
Electronmicroscopy shows the characteristic virus particles in the faecal specimens from these patients.

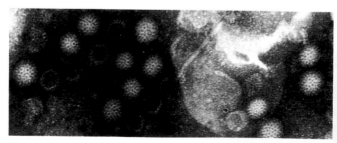

Fig. 73 Electronmicrograph showing rotaviruses. This virus is responsible for a large majority of all cases of infantile gastroenteritis, manifest clinically by diarrhoea and dehydration. The virus particle has a diameter of about 60-65 nm and has the appearance of radial spokes projecting from a central core of double-stranded DNA. x93,800.

Parasitic diarrhoea

Common pathogens: *Entamoeba histolytica*
Giardia lamblia
Intestinal worms

Description
Entamoeba histolytica (Figs. 74 and 75) is the simplest form of unicellular parasite. It causes clinical symptoms varying from mild diarrhoea to acute colitis with ulceration of the gut wall leading to blood-stained faeces containing mucus. From the gut wall these parasites sometimes invade the bloodstream and form metastatic abscesses in various organs including the liver, brain and lung.
Giardia lamblia, also unicellular, is a flagellated parasite of the gut (Figs. 76 and 77). This parasite causes frothy, voluminous diarrhoea with abdominal pain. Prolonged giardial diarrhoea may result in malnutrition resembling tropical sprue syndrome (Fig. 78).
Intestinal worms: various worm infestations may result in mild to severe diarrhoea along with other local (obstructive) and systemic (allergic or migrating) manifestations. Such symptoms are most commonly due to *Ascaris lambricoïdes* (round worm), *Ankylostoma duodenale* (hook worm) and *Taenia* (*solium* and *saginata* - pork and beef tapeworms).

Laboratory study
Microscopic examination of faeces is the most direct method of visualizing the gut parasites. A saline preparation (faeces mixed with a drop of normal saline on a microscope slide) usually allows detection and identification of most of these parasites (by whole or part of the parasite, ova or cyst) in moderate to heavy infestations. A concentration technique improves the rate of detection and is routinely used in the clinical laboratory. The parasites are identified by their typical morphology.

Treatment
Metronidazole is extremely effective in both amoebic and giardial infections.

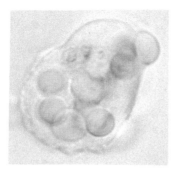

Fig. 74 *Entamoeba histolytica* - trophozoite or vegetative form, found in the acute stage of the disease. The trophozoite often contains ingested red blood cells. *x3,500.*

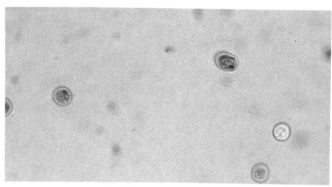

Fig. 75 *Entamoeba histolytica* - cystic form, found in chronic disease and in carriers. Four nucleoli and a chromoidal bar are found within the thick cell wall (Burrow's stain). *x1,000.*

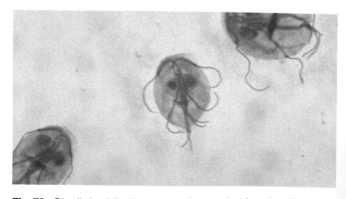

Fig. 76 *Giardia lamblia* - trophozoite (vegetative) form in culture. This form is associated with acute infection in man. *x2,500.*

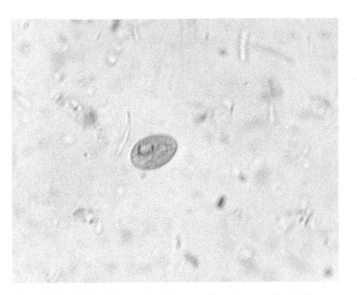

Fig. 77 *Giardia lamblia* - cysts. These are found more often in the chronic form of the disease, characterized by steatorrhoea. *x1,300.*

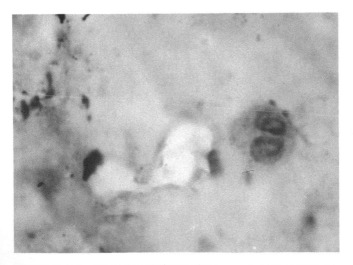

Fig. 78 Trophozoite and cystic forms of the parasites are sometimes found in the jejunal biopsies from cases of malabsorption syndrome. In this figure, a trophozoite form is seen in the biopsy. *x3,000.*

ANAEROBIC INFECTIONS

anaerobic infections	
pathogens	**diseases**
Clostridia (Gram-positive rods)	
Clostridium perfringens (welchii)	gas gangrene, food poisoning
Clostridium tetani	tetanus
Clostridium botulinum	botulism
other Clostridia	minor infections
including *Clostridium difficile*	diarrhoea
Bacteroides (Gram-negative rods)	
Bacteroides fragilis *Bacteroides melaninogenicus* other Bacteroides species	anaerobic septicaemia, lung abscess, deep abscesses e.g. brain abscess
Fusobacteria (Gram-negative rods)	
Fusobacterium necrophorum other Fusobacterium species	various infections including Vincent's angina (in association with *Borrelia vincentii*)

Gas Gangrene
Clostridium perfringens (welchii)

Description
An anaerobic Gram-positive rod (Fig. 79), usually
devoid of spores (cf. other *Clostridia*), this is found
commonly as a commensal in the gut of man and
animals and also in the soil. This organism causes
extensive tissue necrosis with gas formation due to
production of exotoxins, especially α-lecithinase. Infection is usually acquired endogenously from the patient's
own gut flora and is commonly preceded by a relatively
anoxic condition of tissues and in association with a
foreign body. An enterotoxin-producing variety of this
organism (usually heat resistant to 100°C) causes food-
poisoning.

Laboratory study
Culture Necrotic tissue material or exudate from the
infected site produces haemolytic colonies on blood agar
when cultured anaerobically (Fig. 80). Addition of
neomycin or kanamycin to the medium allows pure
isolation (Fig. 81).
Identification The identity of the isolate is confirmed
by its Gram stained morphology (Gram-positive truncated rods without spores), failure to grow aerobically
(some strains can grow slightly) and by the Nagler test
which also confirms the production of the potent α-
lecithinase (Fig. 82).

Antibiotic sensitivity
These organisms are usually very sensitive to penicillin,
metronidazole and erythromycin (Fig. 83), penicillin
being the drug of choice. Treatment includes debride-
ment of necrosed tissue and hyperbaric oxygen in severe
infection.

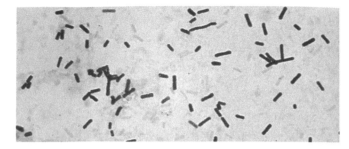

Fig. 79 Gram-positive stout and truncated non-sporing bacillus, *Clostridium perfringens (welchii)*, grown from a gas gangrene lesion. x2,800.

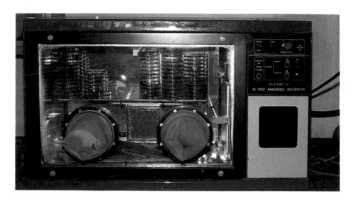

Fig. 80 An anaerobic cabinet which allows isolation of fastidious anaerobes.

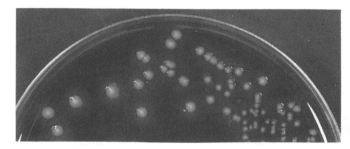

Fig. 81 Pure growth of *Clostridium perfringens* on neomycin blood agar, incubated anaerobically. Most strains produce slight haemolysis. Strains associated with food poisoning are usually non-haemolytic.

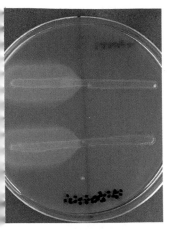

Fig.82 Nagler test-a toxin-antitoxin neutralization test. This test is done on egg-based medium to provide lecithin. *Clostridium perfringens* produces a potent α-lecithinase toxin. This splits lecithin, resulting in visible precipitation around growth. On the other half of the plate, antibody to α-lecithinase is layered, which neutralizes any α-lecithinase produced and no precipitation occurs. This test therefore acts as an identification test for *Clostridium perfringens*.

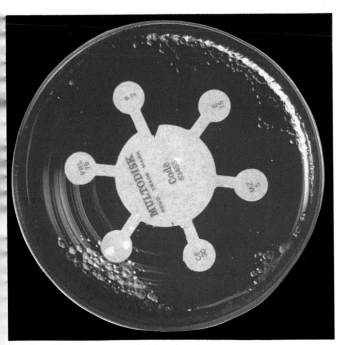

Fig. 83 Antibiotic sensitivity of *Clostridium perfringens*. Usually a wide range of antibiotics are effective against this, including penicillin, erythromycin and metronidazole.

58

Tetanus

Clostridium tetani

Description
A Gram-positive, anaerobic, thin rod-shaped bacillus
with terminal round (drumstick) spore of extremely
potent toxigenic properties (Fig. 84). This is a gut
organism of animals and is also found in soil. The spores
are especially resistant to desiccation and on implant-
ation in human tissue they germinate and produce a
powerful exotoxin. This, on absorption and irreversible
fixation in the nerve cells, causes marked tonic contrac-
tions of the voluntary muscles [due probably to inhibi-
tion of acetyl choline (a neurotransmitter) production at
the inhibitory synapses] resulting in tetani.

Laboratory study
Microscopy and culture Clinical specimens such as
wound exudate show the characteristic microscopic
appearance of the organisms on Gram staining. Anaerobic cultivation of the material on blood agar containing
an antibiotic (neomycin) allows the characteristic thin,
spreading growth of these bacteria with diffuse haemolysis (Fig. 85). Preliminary enrichment of clinical specimens in Robertson's cooked meat medium allows
improved isolation.
Identification This is confirmed by the typical morphology (Fig. 86), colony character and animal pathogenicity (not commonly performed).

Antibiotic sensitivity
These organisms are very sensitive to penicillins, ery-
thromycins and also metronidazole. Anti-tetanus antitoxic serum (preferably human) is essential in the
treatment of clinical tetanus. The toxoid vaccine is
generally used for prophylaxis.

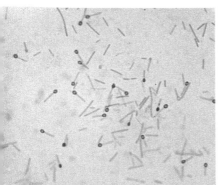

Fig. 84 Gram stained appearance of *Clostridium tetani* showing Gram-positive rods with terminal drumstick spores. *x3,800.*

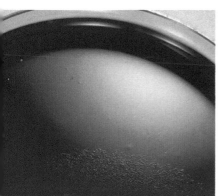

Fig. 85 Growth of *Clostridium tetani*. A thin spreading film, not easily visible to the naked eye, is produced on the surface of the plate. The spreading edge of the film can be seen in this figure.

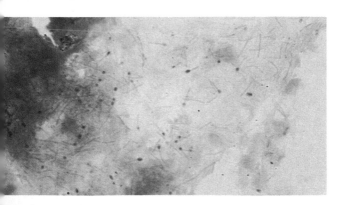

Fig. 86 *Clostridium* spores stained by a special spore staining technique. *x2,500.*

Botulism

Clostridium botulinum

Description
A slender Gram-positive anaerobic bacillus with an oval terminal or subterminal spore, which has the ability to produce the most powerful exotoxin. The toxin, which is heat-labile, is usually produced under strict anaerobic conditions in food, especially canned food, and is absorbed into the bloodstream from the gut on ingestion. After an incubation period of about 20 hours (between 12-72 hours) the clinical manifestations are those of flaccid paralysis of respiratory and voluntary muscles due to blocking of neurotransmission by the toxin at the neuromuscular synapses.

Laboratory study
Culture Culture is not routinely performed, but *Clostridium botulinum* can be cultured from contaminated food. The important diagnostic test is the detection of the presence of toxin in the food by immunodiffusion studies with specific antiserum. An animal pathogenicity test can also determine the lethal property of the toxin. Six antigenic types have been described: types A-F; types A, B and E are more toxigenic than the others.

Antibiotic sensitivity
Antibiotic treatment is not necessary. Antitoxic serum (pooled polyvalent, commercially available) is the mainstay of treatment along with other supportive measures.

Bacteroides infection

Bacteroides fragilis   Bacteroides melaninogenicus
Other *Bacteroides* spp.

Description
These Gram-negative, non-sporing rods are found in
various parts of the body as non-pathogenic commensals (Fig. 87). Bacteroides species, including *Bacteroides fragilis*, constitute the major part of the normal
faecal flora. *B. fragilis* has been implicated as the
commonest pathogen in post-operative infections
related to the gastrointestinal tract, including generalized septicaemia and localized sepsis.

Laboratory study
Culture Clinical specimens transported in anaerobic
transport medium (Stuart) allow isolation of pathogenic
Bacteroides spp., especially *B. fragilis*, using strict
anaerobic procedure (Fig. 88). A pre-reduced blood
agar is a suitable medium for their growth. *Bacteroides
melaninogenicus* produces characteristic black-
pigmented colonies (Fig. 89)
Identification Although biochemical tests are
available for the identification of *Bacteroides* spp., these
are not routinely used. The major volatile fatty acid
pattern shown in gas-liquid chromatography is
employed in some laboratories for their identification.
Colony character, strict anaerobic growth, a Gram stain
and metronidazole sensitivity generally allow easy
identification.

Antibiotic sensitivity
These organisms are uniformly sensitive to metronidazole, the drug of choice for their treatment.

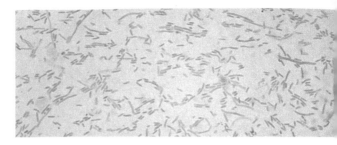

Fig. 87 Gram stained film of *Bacteroides fragilis* showing Gram-negative bacilli with some pleomorphism. *x3,000.*

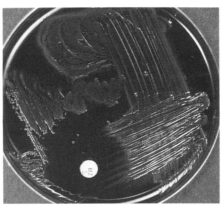

Fig. 88 Culture plate showing growth of *B. fragilis* on blood agar medium incubated anaerobically. A metronidazole disc is implanted for rapid identification. *B. fragilis* is uniformly sensitive to metronidazole.

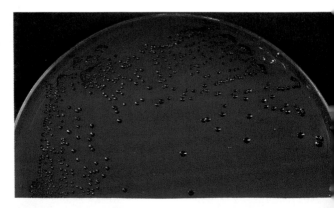

Fig. 89 Growth of *Bacteroides melaninogenicus* showing typical black-pigmented colonies.

Fusobacteria

Fusobacterium necrophorum
Other Fusobacterium spp.

Description
Gram-negative anaerobic rods of variable morphology, some showing a typical fusiform appearance (Fig. 90), while others vary from coccoid to long filamentous forms. They are found as commensals in the mouth and gums of man and animals and also in various necrotic lesions including Vincent's angina in the mouth (Fig. 91), gingival ulcers and lung abscesses.

Laboratory study
Culture These are very fastidious, oxygen-sensitive anaerobes and can be isolated from clinical specimens in well-reduced transport media by the usual anaerobic culture methods (Fig. 92). Microscopic morphology and specialized biochemical tests will identify the organisms.

Antibiotic sensitivity
Fusobacteria are usually sensitive to penicillins, erythromycin, metronidazole and a wide variety of other antibiotics.

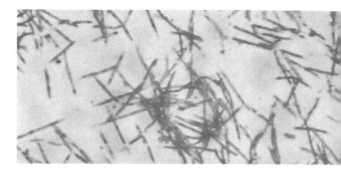

Fig. 90 Gram stained film of *Fusobacterium* sp. showing typical fusiform morphology. *x2,600.*

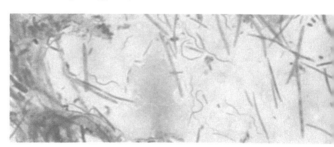

Fig. 91 Gram stained smear of mouth swab from a patient with Vincent's angina. In this, fusobacteria and a spirochaete *Borrelia vincentii* produce a symbiotic combination and cause a very painful gingival infection. This figure shows the cigar-shaped fusiforms with large numbers of spiral *Borrelia*. *x2,500.*

Fig. 92 Growth of *Fusobacterium necrophorum* on blood agar medium.

URINARY INFECTIONS

Common pathogens: *Escherichia coli*
Streptococcus faecalis   *Proteus* spp.
Klebsiella spp.   *Pseudomonas* spp.
Rarely: *Staphylococcus epidermidis*
Staphylococcus aureus   *Streptococcus pyogenes*
Group B streptococcus

Description
Acute infections of the urinary tract could be due to a
multitude of agents. Most urinary infections are ascend-
ing, hence gut organisms are commonly involved; *E. coli*
is responsible for 80% of these infections. Sometimes
the infections are transmitted during surgical manipula-
tions (catheter, cystoscopy etc.). Descending infections
are usually haematogenous - staphylococcus and *Streptococcus pyogenes* are common examples - usually the
source of infection is elsewhere e.g. osteomyelitis.

Laboratory study
A freshly-voided, clean, mid-stream specimen of urine,
cultured on blood and MacConkey's (or CLED) agar
would allow growth of most pathogens. In conjunction
with information from cultures, the presence of RBC,
pus cells, casts and crystals provides clues to the diagnosis (Figs. 93-97). More than 10^5 organisms per ml of
urine is accepted as the threshold of 'significant bacteri-
uria' and is considered to be a definite indication of
infection in association with an increased white cell
count (Figs. 98 and 99).
Identification A significant culture is identified by the
usual biochemical, serological (if applicable) and other
special tests.

Antibiotic sensitivity
An appropriate antibiotic sensitivity test with antibiotics used in the treatment of urinary infection provides guidelines for treatment (Fig. 100). Generally,
urinary infections are amenable to treatment with ampicillin, trimethoprim (or co-trimoxazole), nitrofurantoin
and nalidixic acid (except *Pseudomonas*).

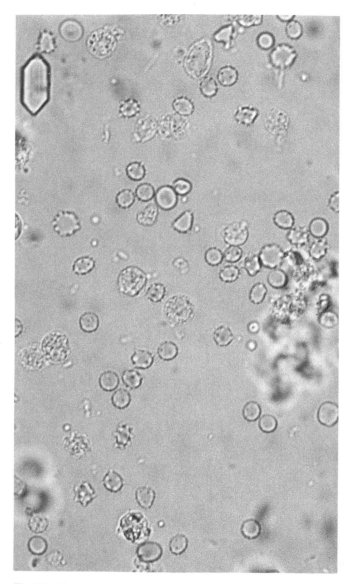

Fig. 93 Microscopy of urine showing presence of pus cells (dead polymorphs), red blood cells and bacteria. This indicates acute infection of the urinary tract. x2,600.

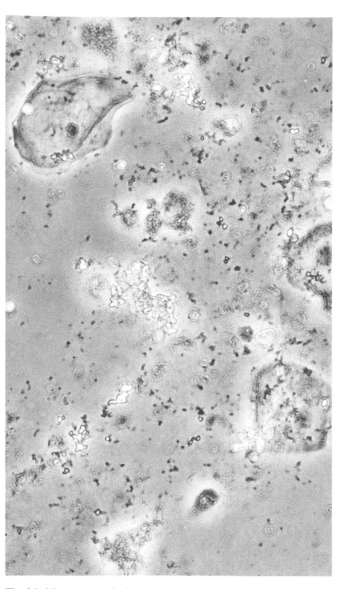

Fig. 94 Microscopy of urine showing a large number of squamous epithelial cells, bacteria and some pus cells. This is improperly collected urine (probably the forepart of urine carrying urethral epithelial cells and bacteria). *x2,600.*

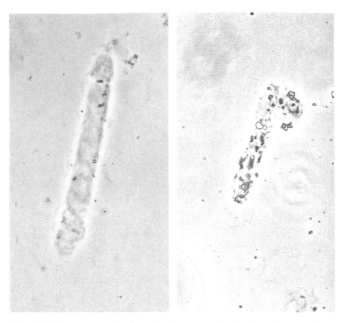

Fig. 95 Microscopy of urine showing a hyaline (left) and a granular cast (right). x1,600.

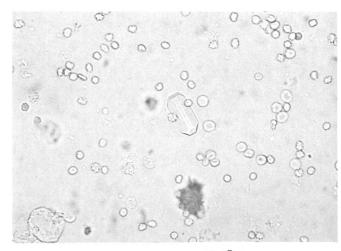

Fig. 96 Microscopy of urine showing coffin-lid shaped phosphate crystals, pus cells and red blood cells. x1,100.

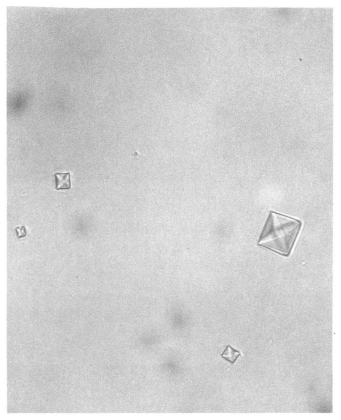

Fig. 97 Microscopy of urine showing calcium oxalate crystals. x1,100.

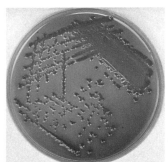

Fig. 98 Pure culture of lactose-fermenting bacteria (*E. coli*) on MacConkey's medium in significant numbers (>300 colonies from one loopful of urine delivering 0.003 ml).

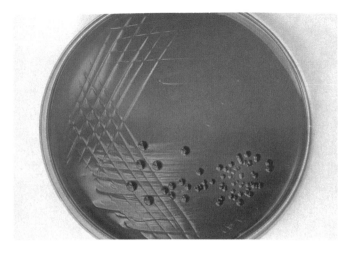

Fig. 99 Pure culture of lactose-fermenting coliform bacteria on MacConkey's medium in insignificant numbers (<100 colonies from one loopful).

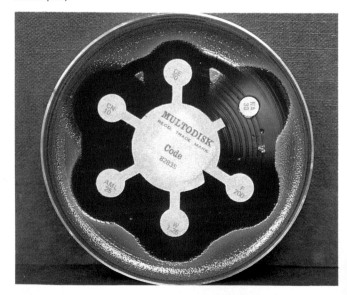

Fig. 100 Antibiotic sensitivity of *E. coli* isolated in significant number from urine. Antibiotics include ampicillin, trimethoprim, nitrofurantoin and nalidixic acid, the four common antibiotics used in urinary infection.

71

INFECTIONS OF THE NERVOUS SYSTEM

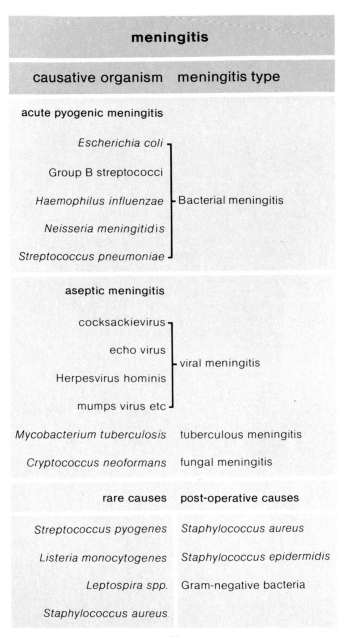

meningitis	
causative organism	**meningitis type**

acute pyogenic meningitis

Escherichia coli	
Group B streptococci	
Haemophilus influenzae	Bacterial meningitis
Neisseria meningitidis	
Streptococcus pneumoniae	

aseptic meningitis

cocksackievirus	
echo virus	
Herpesvirus hominis	viral meningitis
mumps virus etc	
Mycobacterium tuberculosis	tuberculous meningitis
Cryptococcus neoformans	fungal meningitis

rare causes	**post-operative causes**
Streptococcus pyogenes	*Staphylococcus aureus*
Listeria monocytogenes	*Staphylococcus epidermidis*
Leptospira spp.	Gram-negative bacteria
Staphylococcus aureus	

Pyogenic meningitis

Escherichia coli
Group B streptococci } Neonatal meningitis
Haemophilus influenzae   *Neisseria meningitidis*
Streptococcus pneumoniae

Description
This is an acute infection of the meninges and sub-arachnoid space caused by any of the above bacteria. It is characterized clinically by headache, fever, photo-phobia and sometimes loss of consciousness, skin rash and haemorrhages (in meningococcal meningitis), neck rigidity and positive Kernig's sign.

Laboratory study
Culture Cerebrospinal fluid collected by lumbar puncture is transported immediately to the laboratory. A microscopic examination before culture indicates the extent and the nature of exudate: polymorphic or lymphocytic, and also allows visualization of the causative agent on staining (Figs. 101-105). Culture on blood and chocolate agar media will support the growth of the above pathogens (Figs. 106-108). A blood culture at the same time is also likely to yield a positive result. Other media may be included to improve the chances of isolation of additional agents e.g. anaerobic medium for anaerobes and microaerophilic bacteria (in a brain abscess). Changes in the biochemical constituents in the CSF, e.g. decrease in sugar and increase in protein, are useful indications of infections.

Identification Any positive growth from CSF is identified by the usual biochemical, serological and other established methods (Fig. 109). Counterimmuno-electrophoresis (Fig. 110) sometimes helps in the early detection of bacterial antigens in the CSF, particularly when the patient is partially treated.

Antibiotic sensitivity
Appropriate antibiotics like chloramphenicol, ampi-cillin and penicillins are included in the sensitivity testing. In the case of unusual organisms and in neo-natal meningitis, sensitivity testing may need to be extended to include aminoglycosides and other appro-priate antibiotics.

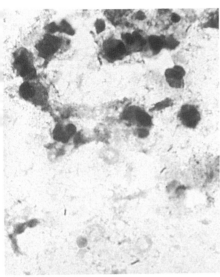

Fig. 101 Gram stained smear of turbid cerebro-spinal fluid from a neonate with meningitis showing pus cells and Gram-negative rods - *E. coli.* x2,800.

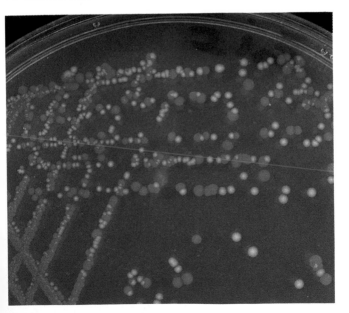

Fig. 102 Growth of group B streptococcus (yellow colonies) from a cervical swab taken from the mother of a neonate who developed group B streptococcal meningitis. The medium is ionagar.

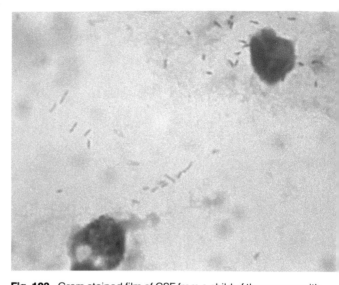

Fig. 103 Gram stained film of CSF from a child of three years with meningitis, showing thin Gram-negative rods which on culture grew *Haemophilus*. x2,800.

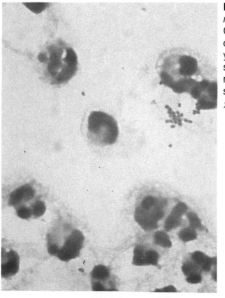

Fig. 104 *Neisseria meningitidis* in a Gram stained smear of CSF from an eleven year old child. The smear shows Gram-negative, bean-shaped diplococci. x3,800.

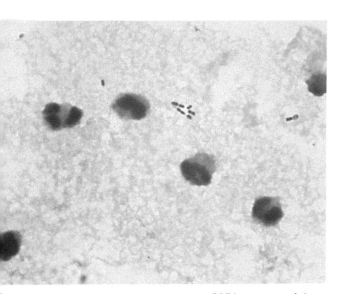

Fig. 105 *Streptococcus pneumoniae* in the CSF from a man of sixty who suddenly became unconscious with signs of meningitis. The smear shows Gram-positive diplococci and pus cells. *x3,400*.

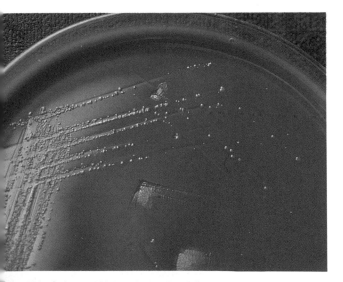

Fig. 106 Culture of *Neisseria meningitidis* on chocolate agar medium.

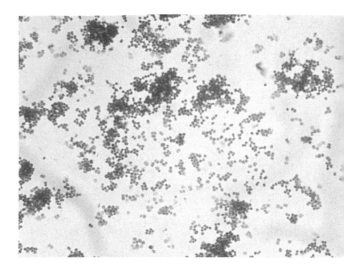

Fig. 107 Gram stained film of *Neisseria meningitidis* showing Gram-negative diplococci. x3,000.

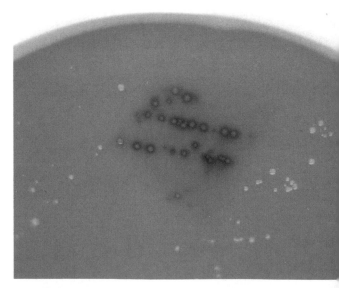

Fig. 108 Oxidase test on *Neisseria meningitidis* on a chocolate agar plate. The colonies turn purple on addition of oxidase reagent and so are oxidase positive. The test can also be done on a filter paper strip as with *Pseudomonas* (see Fig. 39).

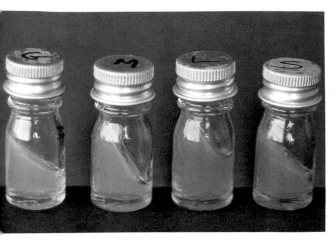

Fig. 109 Sugar fermentation test for *Neisseria*. *N. meningitidis* ferments glucose and maltose, producing acid which changes the colour of the media from pink to yellow. *N. gonorrhoea* ferments only glucose.

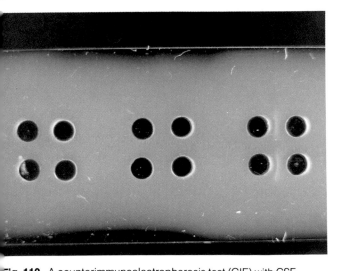

Fig. 110 A counterimmunoelectrophoresis test (CIE) with CSF showing positive precipitation with pneumococcal antiserum, confirming pneumococcal meningitis. Also included in this test are antibodies to *Haemophilus* and meningococcus (negative wells). This test provides rapid diagnosis (30 minutes to 1 hour) and is useful in partially treated cases.

Aseptic meningitis

Viruses - ECHO, mumps, coxsackie (Fig. 111), *Herpes simplex* (Fig. 112)
Bacteria - *Mycobacterium tuberculosis*
Fungus - *Cryptococcus neoformans*

Description

Aseptic meningitis is defined as meningeal infection due to viruses and other agents, in which the CSF remains clear. In virus infections and infections due to mycobacteria and *Cryptococcus*, clinical manifestations are usually mild meningeal irritation and meningism. Tuberculous meningitis can, however, manifest as acute meningitis. Aseptic meningitis due to virus infection is the commonest form of meningeal infection and occurs more commonly in children. In some of these infections the symptoms of meningeal infection merge with symptoms of encephalitis, e.g. herpesvirus infection.

Laboratory study

Culture Microscopic examination shows characteristic inflammatory cells e.g. lymphocytes. An acid-fast stain of spun CSF may show mycobacteria in tuberculous meningitis. CSF culture for viruses can lead to isolation of the virus responsible but is not always possible or required. Serology with paired sera may be useful for retrospective diagnosis. Culture of a faecal specimen often results in isolation of enteroviruses. Isolation of *M. tuberculosis* can be made by routine technique, but pre-enrichment in Kirschner's medium may be helpful. Indian ink preparation of CSF allows direct visualization of the capsulated yeast-like *Cryptococcus* (Fig. 113). Culture on Sabouraud's medium or a richer BHI (brain heart infusion) medium allows isolation of the fungus both at 37° and at 25°C.

Antibiotic sensitivity

Treatment of mycobacterial infection has been dealt with already (page 29). A combination of amphotericin B and flucytosine is an adequate regimen for the treatment of cryptococcal infection. Antiviral agents may be useful in the management of herpesvirus encephalitis.

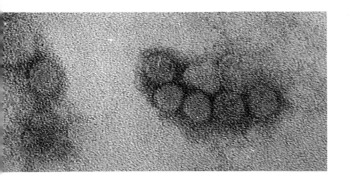

Fig. 111 Electronmicrograph of coxsackievirus: a common agent of viral meningitis. These are very small enteroviruses (about 20-30 nm in diameter) and can be isolated from the throat and faeces of the patient. ECHO virus, another enterovirus of similar morphology is the commonest cause of aseptic meningitis. *x300,000.*

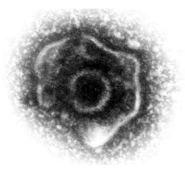

Fig. 112 Electronmicrograph of a herpesvirus showing the typical large envelope around a mature virus particle. *x51,000.*

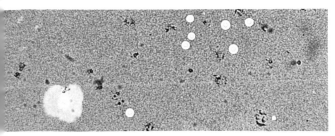

Fig. 113 *Cryptococcus neoformans* in the CSF. An Indian ink preparation showing yeast-like bodies with a large clear capsule. *x1,300.*

SEXUALLY TRANSMISSIBLE AGENTS

Syphilis - *Treponema pallidum*

Description

These are delicate spiral organisms with tapering ends, not affected by ordinary stains but visible under dark ground illumination (Fig. 114) or stained by the silver staining method (Fig. 115). In tissues, the characteristic cork-screw appearances can be seen by using the silver stain. This organism causes an acute infection of the genitalia as a primary infection following sexual contact with an infected partner. This is followed by a more generalized secondary stage including lymphaden-opathy, skin rashes and oral ulcers. In untreated patients, spontaneous healing can occur occasionally. Late manifestations occur in a proportion of cases. These include chronic granulomatous lesions in the liver, brain, bones and large blood vessels.

Laboratory study

Microscopy Serous exudate from primary genital lesions (chancres) shows motile coiling organisms on dark ground microscopy. Pathogenic treponemes are non-cultivable. Serology provides useful information. In active and primary infections, the VDRL (Venereal Diseases Research Laboratory) test - or one of its later modifications like the RPR Card Test (Fig. 116) or APR test and fluorescent treponemal antibody absorption (FTA-Abs) tests (Fig. 117) are usually positive. A positive FTA-Abs IgM test is diagnostic of active disease. In chronic and non-reactive infections and in treated individuals, IgG persists for a very long period and the FTA-Abs IgG test therefore remains positive. The VDRL test can become negative in treated individuals. The TPHA (*Treponema pallidum* haemagglutination) test also detects IgG and can remain positive for a long period. Neither of these tests (FTA-Abs and TPHA) can differentiate between syphilitic infection and other treponemal infections like pinta (*T. carateum*) and yaws (*T. pertenue*) which are found in some parts of the world (West Indies) and are morphologically indistinguishable from *T. pallidum*.

Antibiotic sensitivity

Penicillin is the drug of choice in the treatment of syphilis. Erythromycin and tetracyclines are good alternatives in penicillin-hypersensitive patients.

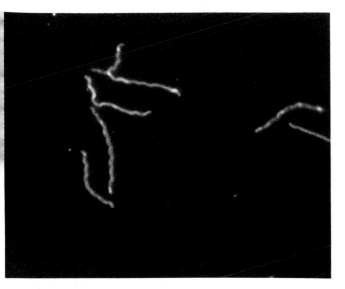

Fig. 114 Dark-ground microscopy of a serous exudate from a genital lesion showing *Treponema pallidum*. x3,300.

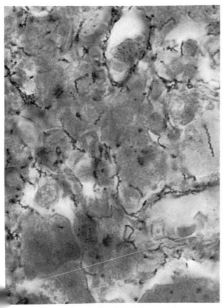

Fig. 115 Silver stain of a section of liver with gummata showing large numbers of darkly-staining, corkscrew-shaped *Treponema pallidum*. x3,000.

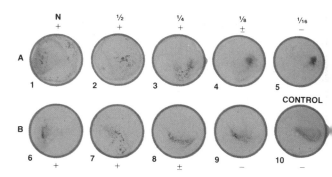

Fig. 116 RPR card test (Rapid plasma reagin) - A VDRL test. Although this test is not very specific, it provides valuable information in the early stages of the disease.

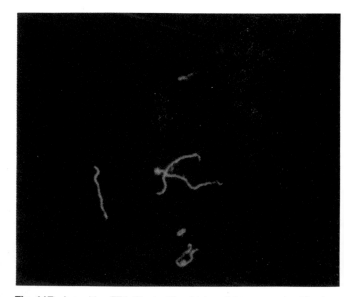

Fig. 117 A positive FTA-Abs test in which anti-treponemal antibody in the patient's blood binds with a dried suspension of *Treponema pallidum*. This complex is then stained with fluorescein-labelled anti-immunoglobulin (IgG or IgM) and is examined under ultra-violet light. x3,600.

Gonorrhoea - *Neisseria gonorrhoeae*

Treat: Cefoxitin /Tetracycline

Description
Neisseria gonorrhoeae is a bean-shaped, Gram-negative diplococcus found predominantly inside pus cells in acute infections. A large number may also be found surrounding the pus cells but the presence of these organisms inside pus cells is diagnostic. (Fig. 118). Infections due to this organism usually start locally (genital organs) but systemic spread is common, involving the epididymis, testes and prostate in the male and the endometrium and tubo-ovarian structures in the female. Blood-borne infections can occur and may sometimes lead to arthritis. The rectum and pharynx may be involved in homosexuals.

Laboratory study
Culture Urethral pus cultured without delay provides positive isolation. As the urethra, particularly in the female, is grossly colonized by gut bacteria, a selective medium (Thayer Martin) containing various antibiotics (blood agar with vancomycin, nystatin, trimethoprim and colistin) allows isolation of this organism in pure culture.

Identification Identification is confirmed by Gram morphology, the oxidase test (see page 24 and Fig. 108) and biochemical tests - a special medium with 1% serum sugar is used. (Fig. 119). Fluorescent antibody staining is also useful to confirm the identity of these organisms (Fig. 120).

Antibiotic sensitivity
Pathogenic *Neisseria* (*N. meningitidis* and *N. gonorrhoeae*) are very sensitive to penicillins. A small population of relatively less sensitive organisms which require a higher dose are now occasionally being isolated. Alternative drugs are co-trimoxazole and spectinomycin.

Social and preventive measures are important in the control of spread.

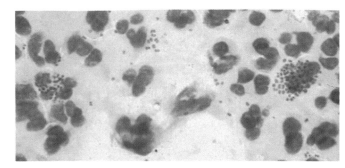

Fig. 118 Urethral pus stained by the Gram method showing a large number of both intra- and extra-cellular Gram-negative diplococci and pus cells. Some pus cells are packed with these organisms. x3,400.

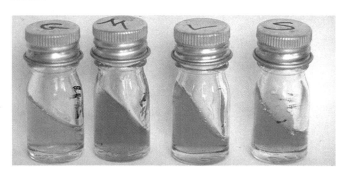

Fig. 119 Sugar fermentation test for *Neisseria*. *N. gonorrhoeae* ferments glucose only and produces acid which changes the colour of the serum-sugar medium from pink to yellow.

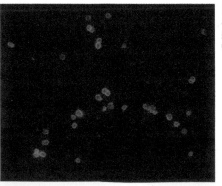

Fig. 120 Fluorescent antibody-stained *N. gonorrhoeae* in urethral pus. x2,800.

Chlamydia trachomatis

Description
These are obligate intracellular parasites sharing characteristics of both bacteria (presence of RNA and DNA, susceptibility to antibacterial antibiotics) and viruses (no cell wall, and failure to grow outside cells). These agents have been incriminated in over half the cases of non-gonococcal urethritis and are a major problem in genito-urinary medicine. *Chlamydia trachomatis* also causes infection in the newborn resulting in inclusion conjunctivitis, as well as deep-seated infection of the female genital tract viz. salpingitis and pelvic inflammatory disease and lymphogranuloma venereum.

Laboratory study
C. trachomatis can be seen in conjunctival scrapings in cases of conjunctival infection (Fig. 121). These can be isolated in tissue cultures and embryonated eggs. Culture is difficult and expensive. A serological test (microimmunofluorescence) is available to detect antibody in the patient's blood as well as for serotyping of the isolates, but this is not performed routinely.

Antibiotic sensitivity
Tetracycline is the most effective antibiotic in the treatment of *C. trachomatis*; erythromycin and minocycline are also effective. Tracing and treatment of contacts and regular follow-up is an important aspect of management.

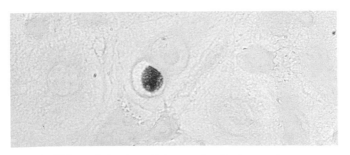

Fig.121 *Chlamydia trachomatis* in a conjunctival smear from a patient with chlamydial ophthalmitis. The slide shows a typical inclusion body stained with iodine. x2,800.

Miscellaneous agents

Gardnerella vaginalis (Haemophilus vaginalis)
Trichomonas vaginalis   *Candida albicans*
Herpes simplex virus - type 2   Hepatitis B virus

Description
The above agents are often isolated from clinical specimens of symptomatic infections from the genitalia in the sexually active age group. Some of these, especially *Gardnerella*, *Trichomonas* and *Candida* produce offensive profuse discharge from the vagina, with vulvovaginal irritation and pain. These are very rarely found in the male but are probably transmitted by men to their sexual partners. Herpesvirus produces single or multiple localized genital ulcerations with involvement of other local tissues including lymph nodes and the epididymis. Hepatitis B is more common in homosexuals (as is hepatitis A).

Laboratory study
Microscopy and culture Both *Trichomonas* (Fig. 122) and *Candida* can be seen in the wet preparation from the transport medium. 'Clue cells' are regularly found in the vaginal discharge in a *Gardnerella vaginalis* infection (Fig. 123). *Candida* and *Gardnerella* can be cultured (Fig. 124 and 125) and identified by their microscopic morphology (Figs. 126 and 127) and biochemical tests. Viruses can be cultured from herpetic lesions and serology confirms the diagnosis of hepatitis B.

Antibiotic sensitivity
In *Gardnerella* infection, there is generally a symbiotic association with anaerobes, and treatment with metronidazole is usually effective; it acts probably by reducing the load of anaerobes. *Trichomonas* is effectively treated with metronidazole, and nystatin applied locally is extremely useful in eradicating *Candida*. Topical ointment containing acyclovir is now available for treatment of genital herpes.

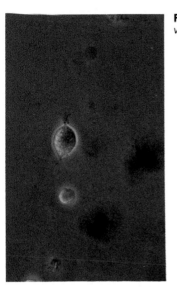

Fig. 122 *Trichomonas vaginalis* in vaginal swab. x1,100.

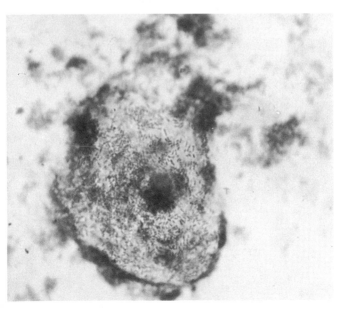

Fig. 123 A 'clue cell'. These cells are characteristically found in vaginal swabs showing epithelial cells heavily colonized with *Gardnerella vaginalis*. x3,700.

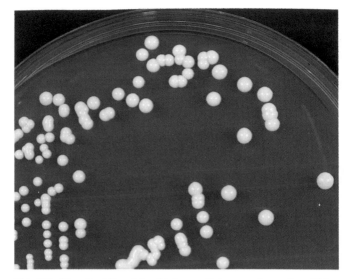

Fig. 124 Growth of *Candida albicans* on Sabouraud's medium. This medium is commonly used for isolation of most fungal agents.

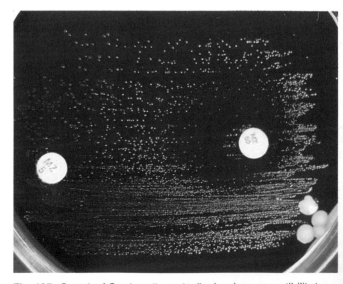

Fig. 125 Growth of *Gardnerella vaginalis* showing susceptibility to a high dose (50 μg) of metronidazole but unaffected by a low dose (5 μg) which is inhibitory to most anaerobes.

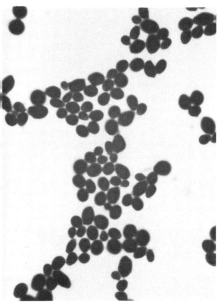

Fig. 126 Gram stained film of *Candida albicans* showing strongly Gram-positive yeast cells of variable sizes. *x3,500.*

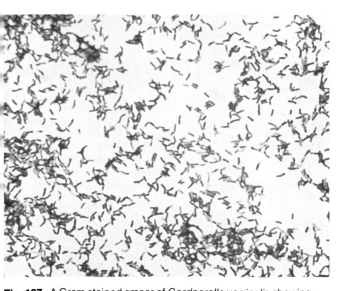

Fig. 127 A Gram stained smear of *Gardnerella vaginalis* showing Gram-variable staining, characteristic of these rod-shaped organisms. *x3,900.*

CUTANEOUS INFECTIONS

Description

A wide range of microbes cause a variety of superficial infections of the skin and subcutaneous tissues. Bacterial infections due to *Staphylococcus aureus* and *Streptococcus pyogenes* are some of the commonest causes and have already been described. Infections by Gram-negative organisms, including anaerobes, occur as secondary invasions on surgical and traumatic wounds and burns e.g. *Pseudomonas aeruginosa* and *Bacteroides fragilis*. *Bacillus anthracis*, a Gram-positive bacillus, usually occurs as an occupational disease in individuals involved in handling contaminated hides and other animal products. Chronic infections due to *Mycobacterium tuberculosis* and *M. marinum* (swimming pool granuloma) are not commonly encountered, but *Mycobacterium leprae* infection (usually of skin) is a major public health problem in many tropical countries (Figs. 128 and 129). Virus infections cause both local skin lesions, as in chickenpox and *Herpes simplex* infections, as well as skin rashes of various types in association with more generalized systemic disease e.g. measles, rubella and mumps.

Superficial fungal infection due to ringworm (dermatophyte) fungus is a common skin disease. *Trichophyton rubrum* and *Microsporum canis* (Figs. 130 and 131) are the two most common skin fungi of man. *Candida albicans* (Fig. 132) is often found in association with mucocutaneous disease.

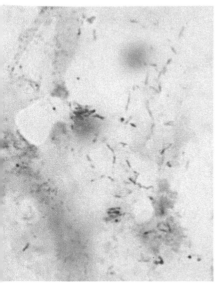

Fig. 128 A Ziehl-Neelson stained film of a slit skin smear from a lepromatous lesion, showing acid-fast bacilli in bundles and small clumps. *x3,100.*

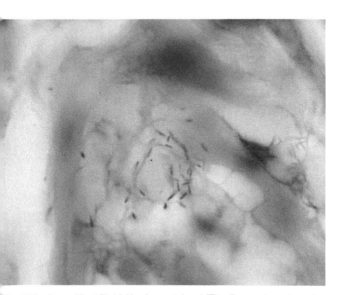

Fig. 129 A modified Ziehl-Neelson stained (Fite-Faraco) section of skin from a patient with leprosy showing large numbers of acid-fast bacilli in the tissues. Some occur in large bundles or globi - a characteristic finding. *x2,800.*

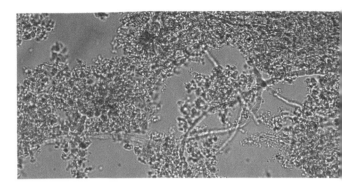

Fig. 130 Fungal hyphae in the skin scraping preparation from a ringworm lesion. The scraped material was treated with 10% KOH and seen under a phase-contrast microscope. *x1,000.*

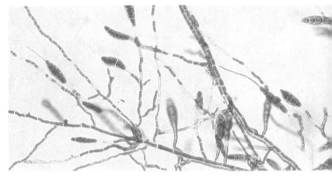

Fig. 131 Spores (macroconidia) and hyphae of *Microsporum gypseum* from a fungal culture stained with lactophenol cotton blue. *Microsporum canis*, a common ringworm fungus, produces similar macroconidia, but these have a tuberculate cell wall. *Trichophyton* species produce numerous microconidia but few macroconidia. Both macro- and microconidia are specialized structures found only under culture conditions. Only hyphae are seen *in vivo*. *x1,100.*

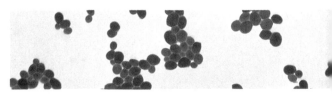

Fig. 132 A Gram stain of *Candida albicans* showing Gram-positive yeast cells. *x2,600.*

SEPTICAEMIA AND PYREXIA OF UNKNOWN ORIGIN

Description
Bacterial and viral infections of the body may be associated with the spread and multiplication of these agents in the bloodstream and are manifested clinically by pyrexia and toxicity. The pyrexia is generally the result of release of toxic microbial products (e.g. endotoxin of Gram-negative organisms) and damaged endogenous cells (e.g. leucocytes). Most bacteria and viruses which cause systemic disease will cause pyrexia. Laboratory support is required for the detection of these microbes. Common bacteria like streptococcus, pneumococcus, *Haemophilus*, *Salmonella* and other Gram-negative bacteria, and viruses like influenza, rubella (Fig. 133), measles (Fig. 134), Epstein-Barr virus – which causes infectious mononucleosis (Fig. 135), poliomyelitis (Fig. 136) and mumps are usually involved as causative agents of pyrexia, but unusual organisms like *Brucella* (Fig. 137), *Leptospira* (Fig. 138), tropical viruses, parasites (Figs. 139-141) and fungi may sometimes be incriminated.

Laboratory study
A thorough history including details of overseas travel and vaccination, and then physical examination will help in deciding the line of investigation. Blood count and culture and other appropriate investigations (e.g. urine culture, X-ray) for bacterial causes and serological tests for virus infections usually provide a definitive answer in most cases within 48-72 hours. In difficult problems, the investigation may need to be extended to include sophisticated and expensive laboratory and other tests e.g. advanced serological and biochemical tests, echocardioradiograph and scanning (using radioisotopes).

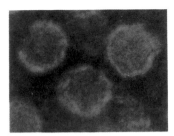

Fig. 133 Electronmicrograph of rubella virus. The virus particle (about 60 nm in diameter) consists of an RNA core surrounded by a rough, ragged envelope. *x224,000*

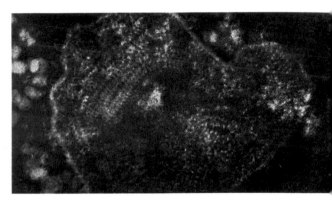

Fig. 134 Electronmicrograph of measles virus. A member of the paramyxovirus family, this is an enveloped RNA virus. It is a common cause of exanthematous disease of childhood. The virus is spread by the respiratory route and causes infection in the throat and upper respiratory tract. Severe infection may result, involving the lower respiratory tract and central nervous system. Serodiagnostic tests and viral isolation in cell cultures confirm the clinical diagnosis. *x194,000*.

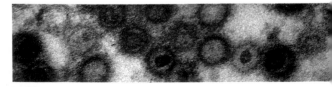

Fig. 135 Electronmicrograph of Epstein-Barr virus (EBV). Morphologically similar to herpesvirus, this virus has a large envelope and a DNA core. During the acute phase of infectious mononucleosis (glandular fever) the virus can be cultured on lymphoblastoid cell lines from the saliva of the patient. Serological tests for heterophile IgM antibodies and the presence of atypical mononuclear cells in the peripheral blood are commonly used diagnostic tests. *x99,000*.

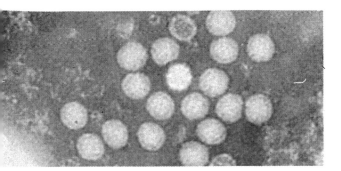

Fig. 136 Electronmicrograph of poliovirus particles. This very small RNA virus (picornavirus) has a particle size of about 20-25 nm in diameter. The small central RNA core is enclosed by protein capsomeres. Other members of the picornavirus family - echoviruses and coxsackieviruses - have a similar morphological structure. ×233,000.

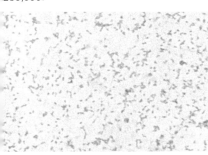

Fig.137 Gram stained film of *Brucella abortus*, showing short, cocco-bacillary, Gram-negative organisms. These are often morphologically indistinguishable from similar organisms such as *Bordetella*. x3,300.

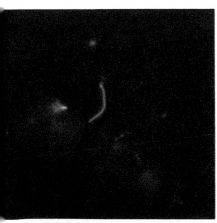

Fig. 138 Dark-ground microscopy used to show *Leptospira*. These spirochaetes are difficult to stain, so dark-ground microscopy or silver staining are usually employed to visualize them. *Leptospira icterohaemorrhagiae* is the most pathogenic species, causing a hepatic necrosis (Weil's disease) which manifests as jaundice with acute toxicity. x2,000.

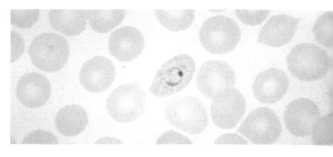

Fig. 139 Giemsa stained blood film from a patient with malaria showing the ring form of *Plasmodium vivax* inside an erythrocyte. *x2,800.*

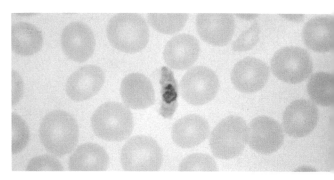

Fig. 140 Giemsa stain of *Plasmodium falciparum* in the peripheral blood showing a crescent-shaped gametocyte. *P. falciparum* cause a malignant or severe form of the disease, sometimes affecting the brain, kidney and other internal organs. *x2,800.*

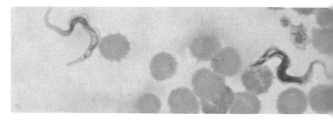

Fig. 141 Giemsa stain of *Trypanosoma* flagellate in a blood smear showing typical morphology. These tissue flagellates cause African sleeping sickness in the sub-Saharan areas of Africa (*T. gambiense* and *T. rhodesiense*), and Chagas' disease, a major public health problem affecting several million patients, in South America (*T. cruzi*) *x2,600.*

OPPORTUNISTIC INFECTIONS

Description
These include infections due to organisms of limited pathogenicity (or even non-pathogenic organisms) occurring in compromised hosts (either immuno-compromised - congenital or acquired, or suffering from prolonged debilitation, due to surgical or medical causes including prolonged drug therapy). Opportunistic infections can cause rapid progressive disease leading to death.

Laboratory study
A wide variety of microbes have been incriminated as opportunistic pathogens including *Pseudomonas aeruginosa* and *Klebsiella*, which are normally not involved in major infections. However, the microbes which have attracted most attention are *Pneumocystis carinii* (Fig. 142), *Toxoplasma gondii* (Figs. 143 and 144), *Cryptosporidium* (Fig. 145), cytomegalovirus (Fig. 146), *Candida albicans* (Fig. 147), *Cryptococcus neoformans* (Fig. 148), *Aspergillus* (Fig. 149), and *Mycobacterium avium-intracellulare* etc. Some of these organisms have been incriminated as being of unusual virulence in immune deficient states like acquired immune deficiency syndrome (AIDS). Specific investigations for most of these agents are available e.g. serological tests for *Pneumocystis*, *Toxoplasma* and cytomegalovirus. Cultural methods are also available for the isolation of some of the common organisms like *Candida albicans*, *M. avium-intracellulare* etc.

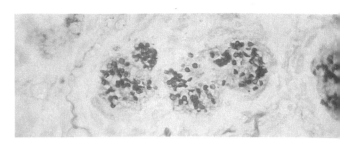

Fig. 142 *Pneumocystis carinii* in lung tissue stained by Grocott modification of methanamine silver-PAS stain. These parasites are found in immunocompromised patients, both during treatment with immunosuppressive drugs as well as in immunodeficiency diseases including AIDS. Diagnosis is difficult and is dependent on the demonstration of the parasites on lung biopsy. Pentamidine iso-thionate treatment shows some benefit. *x3,700*.

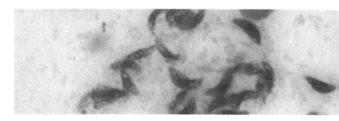

Fig. 143 *Toxoplasma gondii* parasites in Giemsa-stained smear. These parasites cause both mild and severe foetal infections leading to still births or congenital deformities involving the liver, spleen, choroid and retina. Adult infection is usually mild with generalized lymphadenopathy. *T. gondii* also causes severe infections in immunocompromised hosts. Serological tests (toxoplasma dye test) provide evidence of current and past infections. Pyremethamine, co-trimoxazole, sulphonamides and spiramycin have all been used for treatment with variable success. *x2,800*.

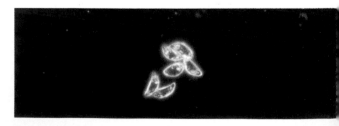

Fig. 144 *Toxoplasma gondii* under dark-ground microscope. *x1,500*.

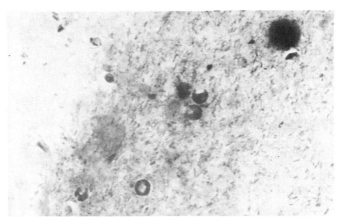

Fig. 145 *Cryptosporidium* - Faeces from a child with diarrhoea stained by the Ziehl-Neelsen method showing *Cryptosporidium* oocysts. These parasites have been found in the faeces of children with self-limiting diarrhoea but their role as a cause of persistent intractable diarrhoea in some immunodeficiency syndromes like AIDS has attracted considerable attention. Treatment so far has remained unsatisfactory. *x2,800.*

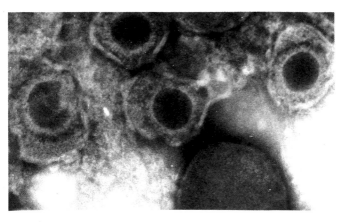

Fig. 146 Electronmicrograph of cytomegalovirus particles. These are morphologically similar to *Herpes simplex* with a diameter of approximately 100 nm and a dense DNA core. Cytomegalovirus is often found in immunosuppresive states, particularly in patients being treated with immunosuppressive drugs (e.g. renal transplant patients) or with cytotoxic agents (e.g. in Hodgkin's disease). Congenital infection in the foetus may result in severe and often fatal illness with involvement of the kidney, liver and spleen. *x126,700.*

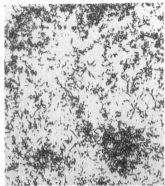

Fig. 147 *Candida albicans* in Gram stain showing polymorphic Gram-positive yeasts. In immunodeficiency conditions, particularly those involving T-lymphocytes, *C. albicans* can cause rapidly developing mucocutaneous granulomatous disease affecting the oral cavity, tracheobronchial tract, vagina and anus. Systemic spread is unusual in the mucocutaneous form of the disease. *x1,500*.

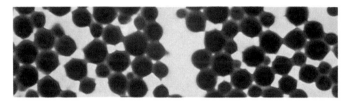

Fig. 148 *Cryptococcus neoformans* culture stained by the Gram method. The film shows yeast-like cells. *C. neoformans* often causes opportunistic infections in immunodeficiency conditions like lymphomas, other T-lymphocyte deficiency diseases, and in patients on prolonged steroid and cytotoxic drug therapy. *x2,600*.

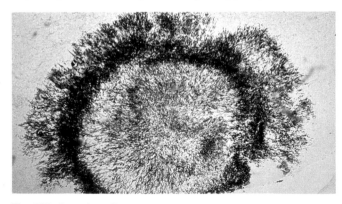

Fig. 149 A section of lung tissue showing invasive aspergillosis on Grocott's methanamine silver-PAS stain. *Aspergillus fumigatus* invasive infections have been reported from various immunodeficiency conditions. *x1,000*.

101

Index